MEDICAL
PARASITOLOGY
A SELF-INSTRUCTIONAL TEXT

EDITION 3

MEDICAL PARASITOLOGY

A SELF-INSTRUCTIONAL TEXT

EDITION 3

RUTH LEVENTHAL, Ph.D., M.B.A., M.T. (A.S.C.P.)
PROVOST/DEAN
PROFESSOR OF BIOLOGY
PENN STATE HARRISBURG
MIDDLETOWN, PENNSYLVANIA

RUSSELL F. CHEADLE, M.S., M.T. (A.S.C.P.)
ASSOCIATE PROFESSOR OF MEDICAL TECHNOLOGY
ASSOCIATE PROFESSOR OF COMPUTER SCIENCE
FLOYD COLLEGE
ROME, GEORGIA

ILLUSTRATIONS BY ELIOT HOFFMAN

F. A. DAVIS COMPANY • Philadelphia

Printed in the United States of America

Last digit indicates print number: 10 9 8 7 6 5 4

NOTE: As new scientific information becomes available through basic and clinical research, recommended treatments and drug therapies undergo changes. The author(s) and publisher have done everything possible to make this book accurate, up-to-date, and in accord with accepted standards at the time of publication. However, the reader is advised always to check product information (package inserts) for changes and new information regarding dose and contraindications before administering any drug. Caution is especially urged when using new or infrequently ordered drugs.

Library of Congress Cataloging-in-Publication Data

Leventhal, Ruth.
    Medical parasitology.

    Includes bibliographies and index.
    1. Medical parasitology—Programmed instruction.
I. Cheadle, Russell F. II. Title. [DNLM: 1. Parasitology—programmed instruction. QX 18 L657m]
QR251.L38   1989   616.9'6'0077   88-31019
ISBN 0-8036-5599-1

To Sheryl, David, Anita, and Bertha—R.L.
To Cathy and Valerie—R.C.

PREFACE TO THE THIRD EDITION

Since the publication of the first edition of *Medical Parasitology,* various social and medical phenomena have increased the incidence of parasitic disease among North Americans. Increased world travel by United States citizens and the recent influx of immigrants to this country from underdeveloped regions, have brought once seldom-encountered parasites to our shores. Changes in sexual behavior have altered the epidemiology of infections such as giardiasis and amebiasis. Finally, the advent of acquired immune deficiency syndrome (AIDS) has unleashed previously rare opportunistic parasites such as *pneumocystis carinii.* Such conditions lend a new urgency to the diagnosis and treatment of parasitic disease by physicians and the detection of these diseases by technologists. We believe, now more than ever, that all health professionals need a fundamental understanding of the diagnosis, treatment, and prevention of parasitic disease. We have approached our revision with this belief in mind.

Medical Parasitology is designed to provide the reader with a concise, systematic introduction to the biology and epidemiology of human parasitic disease. The text is supported throughout by an array of carefully coordinated graphics. Many of the changes incorporated in this revision are based on responses from surveys of the users of the previous editions. The presentation of the symptomatology, pathology, and treatment of each parasitic disease has been expanded. New parasites have been added, most notably those associated with AIDS. Information concerning arthropods' roles as ectoparasites has been enhanced, and coverage of serologic testing has been strengthened.

Enhancements to the graphic elements of the text have not been neglected. One hundred twenty-six captioned color plates are now conveniently located at the front of the text. Eleven new photographs have been added to the chapter on insects. New line drawings have been included and previous drawings modified as necessary. Finally, pedagogical improvements include all new end-of-chapter post-tests and thoroughly updated bibliographies.

Ruth Leventhal
Russell F. Cheadle

ACKNOWLEDGMENTS

The authors particularly wish to thank Dr. Edward D. Wagner of Loma Linda University for his many substantive suggestions. We would also like to thank Ernest J. Davis, D.O., for his extensive review of the text, for his suggestions on drug treatments, and for his contributions to the section on the immunopathology of parasitic infections.

PREFACE TO THE FIRST EDITION

There are many available textbooks about parasitology. Some of these treat the biology of parasites in great depth, while others are more graphic in nature. The laboratorian or clinician needs both kinds. This book was designed to provide a concise description of the biology and epidemiology of human parasites, coupled with an extensive series of color photographs and line drawings to facilitate visual recognition of parasites found in clinical specimens. Furthermore, several modes of graphic presentation have been incorporated in order to aid the various approaches to learning and mastering the requisites.

This book resulted from our recognition of the need for a self-instructional text in parasitology. Present formal course instruction in medical parasitology is often limited and generally is not designed to allow for different learning styles. Russell Cheadle conceptualized and wrote the original draft of this self-instructional text, while the research and writing thereafter became a truly collaborative effort. The product is, we believe, a useful learning tool for students in biology, medical technology, medicine, and public health, as well as an effective pictorial reference book for the clinical laboratory.

We wish to thank Catherine Cheadle, Mary Stevens, and Valerie Fortune for their kind assistance. Russell Cheadle would also like to thank Dr. Herbert W. Cox, his graduate advisor, for his encouragement.

Ruth Leventhal
Russell F. Cheadle

CONTENTS

COLOR PLATES

The series of color photographs included with this text was selected to clearly show you the morphologic and diagnostic characteristics of parasites of medical importance. A brief review of major disease symptoms, the life cycle of the parasite, and other pertinent information are included in the discussion of each photograph. Try to describe each diagnostic stage aloud, recalling the key features of each organism as labeled on the life cycle diagram, to assure yourself that you recall these features.

The Nematoda are a diverse group of roundworms, existing as both free-living and parasitic forms. They vary greatly in size from a few millimeters to over a meter in length. These organisms have separate sexes, and body development is complex. Of the nematode species parasitic for man, about half live as adults in the intestine, and the other half are tissue parasites in their definitive host. The pathogenicity in intestinal infections may be due to biting and blood sucking (e.g., hookworms, *Trichuris*), to allergic reactions caused by substances secreted from adult worms or larvae, or to migration through the body tissues. Tissue nematodes, the Filarioidea, live in various tissue locations in the host. These organisms require an arthropod intermediate host in their life cycle. The pathology produced varies with the location of the parasites in man but may involve the occlusion of the lymphatics (*Wuchereria, Brugia*), localized subcutaneous swellings or nodules (*Onchocerca, Dracunculus*), or blindness (*Onchocerca*).

1,2. *Enterobius vermicularis* (pinworm). 1. Adult male (20×) and 2. female (10×). These mature in the anterior portion of the colon. The adult female worms are 8 to 13 mm and the male worms 2 to 5 mm in size. Each has a bulbar esophagus as well as finlike projections, called cephalic alae, about the anterior end. Male and female worms are further differentiated in that the male has a sharp curvature of the tail and small posterior copulatory spicule, whereas the female has a long, straight, sharply pointed tail. When the uterus is gravid with eggs, the female migrates from the colon (usually during sleeping hours of the host) to the perianal area where she deposits her eggs and dies. Pinworm disease is essentially an allergic reaction to the release of eggs and other secreted materials from the gravid female, which causes severe rectal itching.

3. A higher-power view of the anterior end of the adult, clearly showing the alae.

4. Note the caudal curve and copulatory spicules of the male *Enterobius vermicularis*.

5. *Enterobius vermicularis* eggs (400×). Eggs may be recovered from the perianal folds by applying the sticky side of cellophane tape to the skin surfaces and then taping the cellophane, sticky side down, on a microscope slide for examination. Eggs are rarely recovered in feces. The eggs are elongated (55 μm × 25 μm) and tend to be flattened on one side. The thick shell is transparent and colorless, and the folded larva may be seen within. Pinworm eggs are infective for the host within a few hours of being released. Scratching of the perianal region allows transfer of the eggs to the mouth of the host. The eggs hatch soon after they are swallowed and develop to mature worms within two weeks. Bedding, night clothing, and even house dust may be sources of egg infection for others through ingestion or inhalation of eggs. This is a very common parasitic infection in this country and spreads easily, so that those living with an infected individual are likely to become infected.

6. *Enterobius vermicularis* egg (900×). This view shows an egg under oil immersion; the developed larva can be clearly seen coiled inside the flattened shell.

7. *Enterobius vermicularis* egg (100×). A low-power view of the egg as seen on a cellophane tape preparation. Because of the transparency of the eggs, screening of the slides must be carefully performed, using low illumination.

8. *Trichuris trichiura* (whipworm) (4×). Adult female, measuring 35 to 50 mm. The anterior ends of both male and female worms are slender and threadlike, but the posterior ends are wider. The posterior end of the female appears club shaped and straight; the male has a coiled posterior with two copulatory spicules. The adults in the intestine attach firmly by embedding a spearlike projection at their anterior end into the mucosa of the cecum and proximal colon. Distribution of this parasite is cosmopolitan, especially in moist, warm areas. This is the most commonly reported parasitic infection in this country. Light infections are usually asymptomatic, but heavy infections may cause enteritis and diarrhea with rectal prolapse.

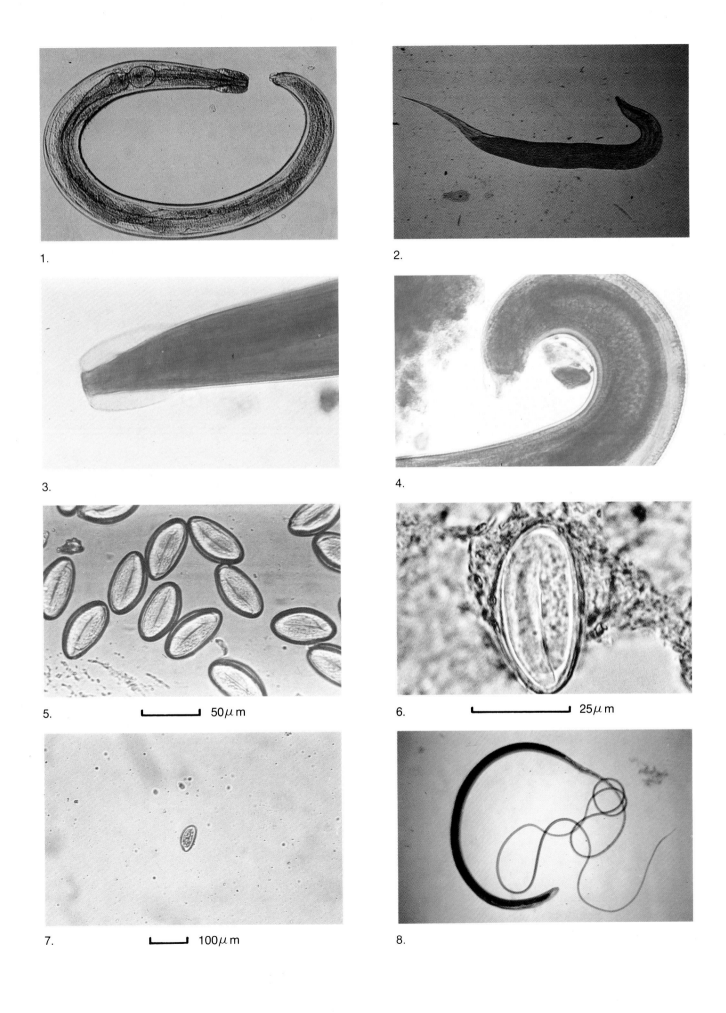

1.

2.

3.

4.

5.　　　　　　　　⊢——⊢ 50μm

6.　　　　　　　　⊢——⊢ 25μm

7.　　　　　⊢—⊢ 100μm

8.

9. *Trichuris trichiura* egg (500×). Diagnosis: recovery of eggs in feces. The *Trichuris* egg is characteristically barrel shaped and measures 20 μm × 50 μm. Note the undeveloped embryo; the clear, inner shell; the heavy, golden outer shell; and the transparent hyaline plugs at the ends of the egg. Eggs passed in feces must remain in a favorable soil environment for at least 10 days until larval development is complete; at this time the egg is infective. Ingestion of the egg from infected soil or contaminated food is followed by hatching in the intestine. The larva molts and develops in the intestines to become an adult. About 90 days are needed for a complete cycle from egg ingestion to egg output by the adults.

10. *Trichuris trichiura* egg. This view shows an egg at a magnification of 100×.

11. *Ascaris lumbricoides.* Both male and female adults are shown. They are conically tapered at the anterior end. A female measures 22 to 35 cm in length by 3 to 6 mm in diameter and has a straight tail. A male measures 10 to 31 cm by 2 to 4 mm and has a sharply curved tail with two copulatory spicules. The adults live in the small intestine and can survive for over a year. Females lay up to 200,000 eggs per day which are passed in the feces and can be recovered by routine fecal examination. Passage of adult worms from the rectum is often the first indication of infection. Light infections are asymptomatic. Heavy infections may cause pneumonia early in the infection and, later, diarrhea, vomiting, or bowel obstruction. Complications such as perforation of the intestinal wall or appendix with resultant peritonitis, or obstruction of airways by vomited worms, may cause death. Known as the large intestinal roundworm.

12. An obstructed bowel from a heavily infected patient. Distribution of this parasite is worldwide, although it is more frequently found in tropical areas.

13. *Ascaris lumbricoides* egg (400×). Diagnosis: recognition of eggs (or adults) in feces. The fertilized egg measures 40 μm × 55 μm and contains an undeveloped embryo. This egg appears round, but *Ascaris* eggs are slightly oval. The outer coat is albuminous and mammillated; occasionally, eggs without coats may be found (decorticated). The inner coat is of clear chitin. These characteristics are diagnostic. On reaching warm, moist soil, larvae develop within the egg shells in 2 to 3 weeks, and eggs are then infective for man. Infection occurs by ingestion of these infective eggs in contaminated food or drink. It is not uncommon for *Ascaris* and *Trichuris* to coexist in the same person because of the method of infection and the requirements for egg development. Eggs hatch in the intestine, and the *Ascaris* larvae rapidly penetrate the mucosal wall. They reach the liver and then the lungs via the blood circulation. Larvae emerge from the circulation into the lungs, migrate up the bronchi to the esophagus, and are swallowed. They mature in the intestine in about 2 months. In an immune individual, most larvae are destroyed in the liver.

14. *Ascaris lumbricoides* egg. This view shows an egg at a magnification of 100×. Ascarids of dogs and cats (*Toxocara* spp.) can undergo partial development and produce pathology in humans. After ingestion, the *Toxocara* egg hatches, and the larvae penetrate the intestinal wall and enter the blood circulation but are unable to complete the migratory route. They lodge in tissues and cause inflammatory reactions leading to occlusions of capillaries of vital organs (e.g., eye, liver, brain, lungs). Symptoms vary depending on the location of the parasite and the host's reaction to it. The disease is called visceral larval migrans. It is seen most commonly in children because they are more likely to ingest eggs from infected soil, such as at a playground where dogs are walked. High eosinophilia is a very common sign. Diagnosis is made serologically or by observing larvae in histopathologic sections. Species identification is difficult but can be done.

15. *Ascaris lumbricoides* egg (400×). An unfertilized egg. Note the elongated shape and the heavy albuminous coat. This type of egg is not uncommonly seen.

16. Adult male hookworm (10×). Adult hookworms are small, grayish-white nematodes. The anterior end is tapered and curved. Females (12 mm × 0.5 mm) are larger than males (9 mm × 0.4 mm). The female has a straight and pointed tail and produces 5,000 to 10,000 eggs per day. She may live up to 14 years. The posterior end of the male terminates in a fan-shaped copulatory bursa and spicules. The raylike pattern of the chitinous supportive structure in the bursa is different for each species.

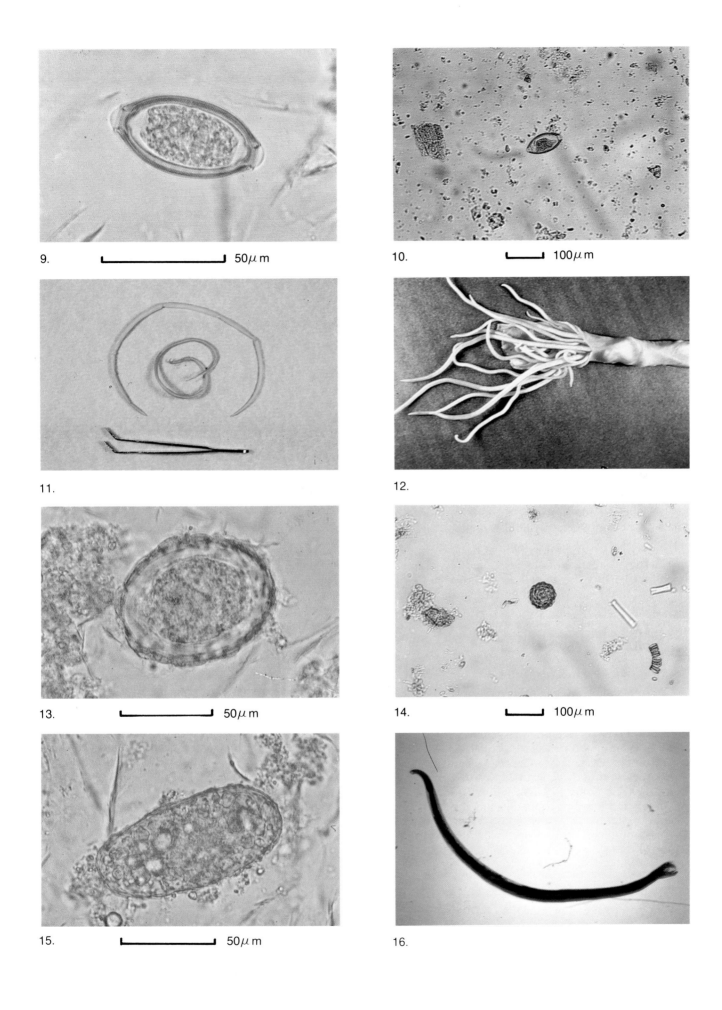

9.   ⊢━━━━━━━━┤ 50μm

10.   ⊢━━┤ 100μm

11.

12.

13.   ⊢━━━━┤ 50μm

14.   ⊢━━┤ 100μm

15.   ⊢━━━━┤ 50μm

16.

17. *Necator americanus* (New World hookworm). The anterior end of an adult worm. Species identification is helped by examining the mouthparts. Note the *pair of semilunar cutting plates* in the upper side of the buccal cavity.

18. *Ancylostoma duodenale* (Old World hookworm). The anterior end of an adult worm. Note the two pairs of teeth in the buccal cavity. The mouthparts of hookworms allow for firm attachment to the mucosa of the small intestine. *N. americanus* is found throughout West Africa and the southeastern United States; *A. duodenale* is found in Europe and the Mediterranean countries. Both are found in parts of Asia, Central and South America, and the South Pacific. Symptoms of the disease depend on the extent of the infection and the nutritional status of the patient and can appear clinically as a hypochromic microcytic anemia because of the blood-sucking activity of worms.

19. Hookworm egg (500×). Note the definite but thin shell and the clear area around the undeveloped larva. Diagnosis of the presence of hookworms may be made upon recognition of the egg in feces, but adults must be examined for species identification because the eggs of these worms look alike. Only a heavy infection causes the disease state. Eggs usually contain an immature embryo in the 4-to-8-cell stage of division if feces are promptly examined. Six cells are visible in this embryo. Eggs measure about 30 μm × 50 μm.

20. Hookworm eggs (500×). This view shows more mature eggs containing developing rhabditiform larvae. Eggs are shed in feces, and the embryo rapidly develops to a larva in 1 to 2 days. Eggs hatch to liberate rhabditiform larvae which then further mature in the soil to become infective filariform larvae.

21. Hookworm rhabditiform larva, showing the anterior end of the first stage larva (500×). Although these larvae are not normally seen in fresh fecal preparations, larvae may develop and hatch if feces are not promptly examined. This view has been included so that differential characteristics between hookworm larvae and *Strongyloides stercoralis* rhabditiform larvae may be studied. Note that the buccal cavity of a first-stage hookworm larva is slightly longer than the width of the head, appearing as two parallel lines extending back from the anterior edge of the larva. It has a longer buccal cavity than that of *S. stercoralis* and is the primary characteristic differentiating the two (see Plate 25). The hookworm larva measures 250 μm × 17 μm.

22. Hookworm filariform larva (100×). Infection occurs when infective stage (filariform) larvae penetrate skin, especially between the toes. The larvae are carried throughout the body via lymphatic and blood circulation. Most larvae emerge from the circulation in the lungs, migrate up the bronchi to the esophagus, and are swallowed. They complete maturation in the intestine in about 2 weeks. Nonfeeding infective hookworm larvae are ensheathed and have pointed tails. A short esophagus extending about one quarter of the way down from the anterior end is another differentiating characteristic.

23. Infective larvae of dog and cat hookworms, especially *Ancylostoma braziliense,* can invade human skin, producing an allergic dermatitis called creeping eruption or cutaneous larval migrans. Inasmuch as man is an unnatural host for the animal hookworms, further larval development does not occur. An itching red papule is produced at the site of larval entry with development of a serpentine tunnel between the epithelial layers produced as the larva migrates. The larva moves several millimeters per day and may survive several weeks or months. This disease is widely distributed and is common in sandy areas on the Atlantic coast from New Jersey to the Florida Keys, along the Gulf of Mexico, and in many parts of Texas. It is also found in the midwestern United States.

24. *Strongyloides stercoralis* (threadworm) (400×). This view is of a rhabditiform larva (225 μm × 15 μm) seen in feces. The esophageal bulb is evident at the junction of the esophagus and intestine, which is about one fourth of the parasite's length back from the anterior end. This is one diagnostic feature that may be used to differentiate hookworm and *Strongyloides* rhabditiform larvae, because this structure is not as prominent in hookworm larvae. Adult parthenogenic female worms (2.2 mm × 50 μm) live in the submucosa of the upper small intestine. Eggs pass through the mucosa, and the rhabditiform larvae hatch in the lumen of the intestine to be shed in feces. The larvae may develop in soil to become infective filariform larvae and penetrate the skin as do hookworm larvae. They may also molt and become infective before they pass in feces and penetrate the mucosa of the colon to cause autoinfection. In either case, they travel via the blood–lung route as do hookworm larvae, returning to the intestine to develop into adults. The life cycle of this parasite may include a free-living cycle in the soil. In this case, rhabditiform larvae molt and develop to become free-living mature adults. The sexually mature free-living male and female mate and produce eggs which develop into filariform larvae which are infective to man via skin penetration.

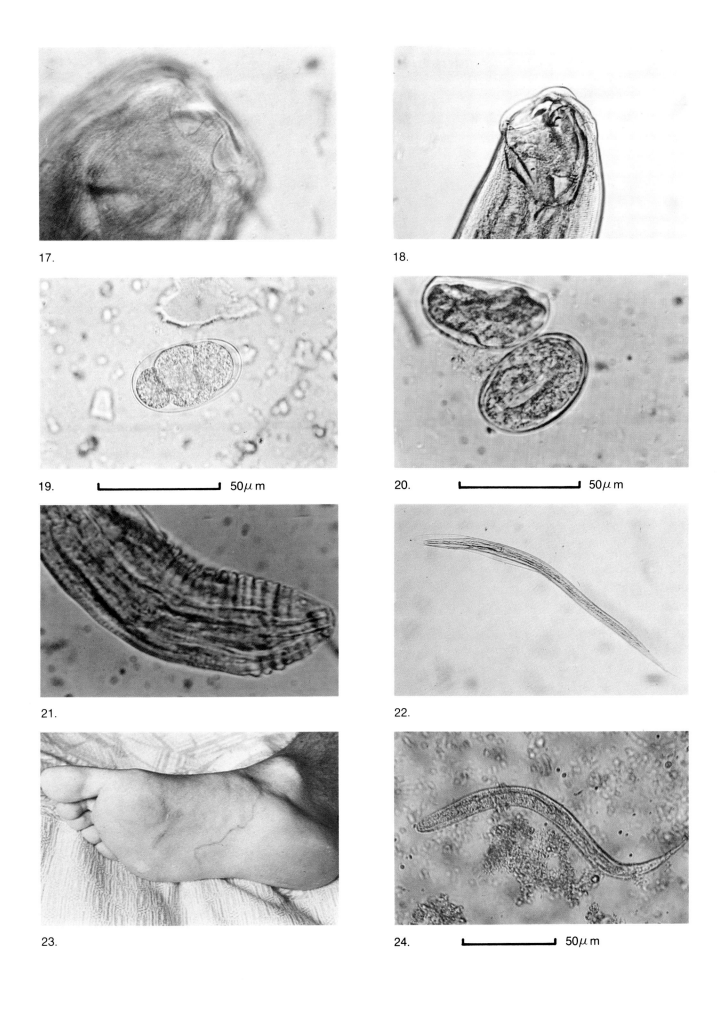

17.

18.

19. |⊢——————⊣| 50μm

20. |⊢——————⊣| 50μm

21.

22.

23.

24. |⊢——————⊣| 50μm

25. *Strongyloides stercoralis* (500×). This view shows the short buccal cavity of the rhabditiform larva. The length is one third to one half the width of the head of the larva (compare with Plate 21). Diagnosis is based on the recovery of characteristic rhabditiform larvae from feces. The filariform (infective stage) larva of *Strongyloides* has a notched tail, whereas the filariform larvae of hookworms have pointed tails. This parasite is found worldwide, especially in warm climates. As with hookworm disease, there is a dermatitis at the site of repeated larval entry, and respiratory symptoms may result from the larvae as they migrate through the lungs. Abdominal symptoms vary with the extent of the infection from mild epigastric pain to vomiting, diarrhea, and weakness with weight loss. Moderate eosinophilia is common. Untreated, the disease may last for many years because of autoinfection from larvae that develop in the colon and may cause death in the immunosuppressed patient.

26. *Trichinella spiralis* (trichina worm). Encysted larva in muscle tissue (400×). Adult worms develop in the submucosal tissues of the small intestine. They are very small: the male measures 1.5 mm, and the female measures 3.5 mm. Larvae produced by the female pass into the mesenteric venules or lymphatics and are carried throughout the body. Within about 2 weeks they emerge from the blood to enter striated muscle cells or other tissue but survive only if they enter striated muscle cells. These are encysted and calcify over time but remain alive for years. Many hundreds of larvae may be produced over the female's life span of 2 to 3 weeks. Infection occurs when undercooked pork or bear meat containing encysted larvae is ingested, and the larvae develop into adults in the intestine in a few days. The disease (trichinosis) is found worldwide among meat-eating populations and presents a variety of symptoms, including gastric distress, fever, edema (especially of the face), and acute inflammation of muscle tissue. Daily study of blood smears showing increasing eosinophilia is a useful diagnostic aid. A history of eating undercooked meat, skin testing, and positive serologic tests are strongly suggestive of infection but are not conclusive. Definitive diagnosis depends upon demonstration of the encysted larvae in a muscle biopsy from the patient. Attempts at recovery of adult parasites from feces are usually futile.

27. *Trichinella spiralis.* A higher-power view of a stained section. Note the tissue inflammation around encysted muscle larvae.

28. *Wuchereria bancrofti* (Bancroft's filaria) microfilaria (400×). A thick peripheral blood smear, stained with Giemsa stain, showing the sheathed embryo, which measures 250 μm in length. The ends of the sheath appear almost colorless and are noncellular. The presence of a sheath and the pattern of cell nuclei, which can be seen in the posterior end of the microfilaria (upper center photograph), are diagnostic. Microfilariae are most prevalent in the peripheral blood at night (nocturnal periodicity); therefore, they are best detected in blood specimens obtained at this time. Adult nematodes live in the lymphatics. Prolonged infections cause obstruction of lymph flow, resulting in elephantiasis of the lower extremities, genitalia, or breasts. Other symptoms include fever and eosinophilia caused by allergic reactions to the parasite. *Culex, Aedes,* and *Anopheles* mosquitoes serve as intermediate hosts of *W. bancrofti* and are found in tropical areas worldwide. Diagnosis: recovery of characteristic microfilariae in blood.

29. *Brugia malayi* (Malayan filaria) sheathed microfilaria (400×). Note that the nuclei occur in groups to the end of the tail (middle right of photograph). These features are diagnostic. The disease produced is essentially identical to *W. bancrofti* but is found primarily in Southeast Asia, India, and China. These microfilariae also exhibit nocturnal periodicity in the blood, and the mosquito vectors are species of *Mansonia* and *Anopheles.* Diagnosis: recovery of characteristic microfilariae in blood.

30. *Loa loa* (eyeworm) microfilaria (400×). In this thick blood smear, the sheathed microfilaria can be seen, measuring 250 μm in length. Note that cell nuclei occur in groups through most of the body but are seen in a single line at the posterior end of the tail (upper right of photograph). This feature is diagnostic. Adults migrate throughout the subcutaneous tissues in man, causing transient swellings called Calabar swellings. Adults may be seen migrating through the conjunctiva of the eye. Microfilariae are most prevalent in the blood during the day (diurnal periodicity), and the vector is the mango fly *(Chrysops).* The disease is chronic and relatively benign, although allergic reactions may occur, causing edema, itching, and eosinophilia. This parasite is found in West and Central Africa. Diagnosis: recovery of characteristic microfilariae in blood.

31. Children with distinct fibrous nodules on their bodies, which contain adult worms of *Onchocerca volvulus.* The female discharges microfilariae that migrate through the skin but do not reach the blood. The disease is chronic and nonfatal. Allergic reactions to microfilariae cause local symptoms. If microfilariae reach the eye, blindness may occur. This parasite is a major cause of blindness in Africa. Diagnosis is made by excising a nodule with recovery of adult worms or by detecting microfilariae in a tissue scraping of the nodule. When present in the eye, microfilariae may be observed with an ophthalmic microscope. The vector is the blackfly, *Simulium,* which breeds in running water, and the disease is found in southern Mexico, Guatemala, Venezuela, and parts of Africa.

32. *Onchocerca volvulus* microfilaria (100×) present in a tissue scraping of a skin nodule.

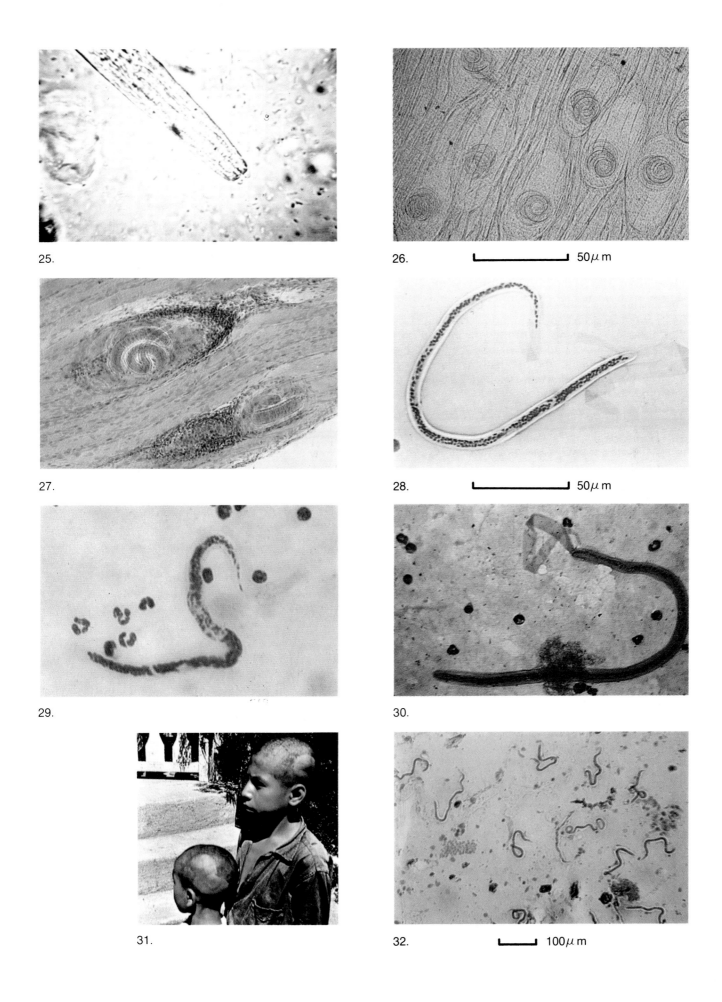

25.

26.　⊢————————⊣ 50μm

27.

28.　⊢————————⊣ 50μm

29.

30.

31.

32.　⊢————⊣ 100μm

33. *Dracunculus medinensis* (Guinea worm). This view shows part of a female worm protruding from an ulcer and wrapped around a match stick. The female is 70 to 120 cm × 2 mm in length. These worms release larvae into water. Infection occurs when man drinks water containing crustaceans of the genus *Cyclops* (the intermediate host) infected with larvae of *D. medinensis.* Larvae liberated from the copepod in the human small intestine migrate through the viscera to the subcutaneous tissues and become adults. In the subcutaneous tissues, the female induces an ulcer and releases larvae into water. Larvae released into fresh water penetrate the intermediate host. The major clinical manifestation of this disease includes allergic symptoms, that is, fever, diarrhea, nausea, eosinophilia, and local symptoms caused by ulcer formation. This parasite is found in the Middle East, Central Africa, the West Indies, and the Guianas. Species that parasitize animals have been found in North America. Diagnosis: detection of the adult in local lesions.

The Cestoda are a subclass of endoparasitic Platyhelminthes (flatworms); the cestodes are commonly known as the tapeworms. The adults live in the intestinal tract of vertebrates, while larval forms inhabit tissues of vertebrates or invertebrates. The head (scolex) is modified by suckers and sometimes hooks for attachment to the intestinal wall, and the segments (proglottids) containing both male and female sex organs bud from the posterior end of the scolex to form the body of the tapeworm (the strobila). The length of tapeworms varies from 2 to 3 mm up to 10 meters. Infection in man produces primarily intestinal symptoms. Transmission to man occurs when insufficiently cooked food containing larvae is eaten or when eggs are ingested.

34. *Hymenolepis nana* (dwarf tapeworm) egg (400×). Diagnosis: recovery of characteristic eggs in feces. Note the threadlike filaments that radiate from two polar thickenings into the area between the embryo and outer shell. Three pairs of hooklets may be seen on the embryo inside the inner shell. Infection is by ingestion of the egg, which hatches in the duodenum. The embryo penetrates the mucosa where it matures to a cysticercoid larva in the intestinal wall. The larva emerges in a few days and develops to an adult worm. No separate intermediate host is required.

35. *Hymenolepis nana* egg (100×). A low-power view of another egg.

36. *Hymenolepis nana* mature proglottids (100×). The proglottid contains a bilobed ovary and three round testes. The testes are visible, but the ovary is not easily seen in this view. Segments usually disintegrate in the intestine before passage in the feces. The whole worm measures 2.5 to 4.0 cm and is the smallest tapeworm to parasitize man. Multiple infections are common, because eggs can hatch in the intestinal tract and cause an immediate autoinfection as the larvae enter the mucosa. The body of the worm (the strobila) contains about 200 proglottids. Each of these flattened segments contains complete male and female reproductive organs. All nutrient is absorbed from the intestine of the host through the tegument of the tapeworm.

37. *Hymenolepis nana* scolex (100×). Four suckers and a retractable rostellar crown with one row of 20 to 30 hooklets. These structures provide for firm attachment to the intestinal mucosa. Light infections may be asymptomatic, but heavy infections produce diarrhea, vomiting, weight loss, and anal irritation. This parasite is found in India and South America and is common in children in the southeastern United States. Autoinfection may occur if eggs hatch inside the host, but usually reinfection is caused by hand-to-mouth transfer from scratching the irritated anal region.

38. *Taenia* species. *Taenia solium* (pork tapeworm) or *Taenia saginata* (beef tapeworm) egg (400×). *Taenia* eggs are diagnostic for the genus only. Notice the thick outer shell with its radial striations. The hexacanth embryo inside the egg shell bears six chitin hooklets. The six hooklets are not visible in this view. Eggs of *T. solium* are infective for both pigs and man. If eggs are accidentally ingested by man, they hatch, just as they do in pigs, in the small intestine. Larval forms *(Cysticercus cellulosae)* develop in the subcutaneous tissues, striated muscles, and other tissues of the body. Symptoms vary with the location of the cyst. Eggs of *T. saginata* are not infective for man. The source of human infection with the adult tapeworm is ingestion of insufficiently cooked pork or beef containing encysted larvae. After being digested free, the scolex of the cysticercus everts and attaches to the small intestine, and the larva grows to become an adult in 6 to 10 weeks.

39. *Taenia* spp. eggs (100×). This view shows four eggs at low power.

40. *Taenia solium* (pork tapeworm) scolex (100×). Four suckers and a rostellum containing 20 to 30 hooklets are set in two rows at the anterior end of the scolex. *T. saginata* can be differentiated from *T. solium* because its scolex does not have hooklets, only four suckers, and is therefore said to be unarmed.

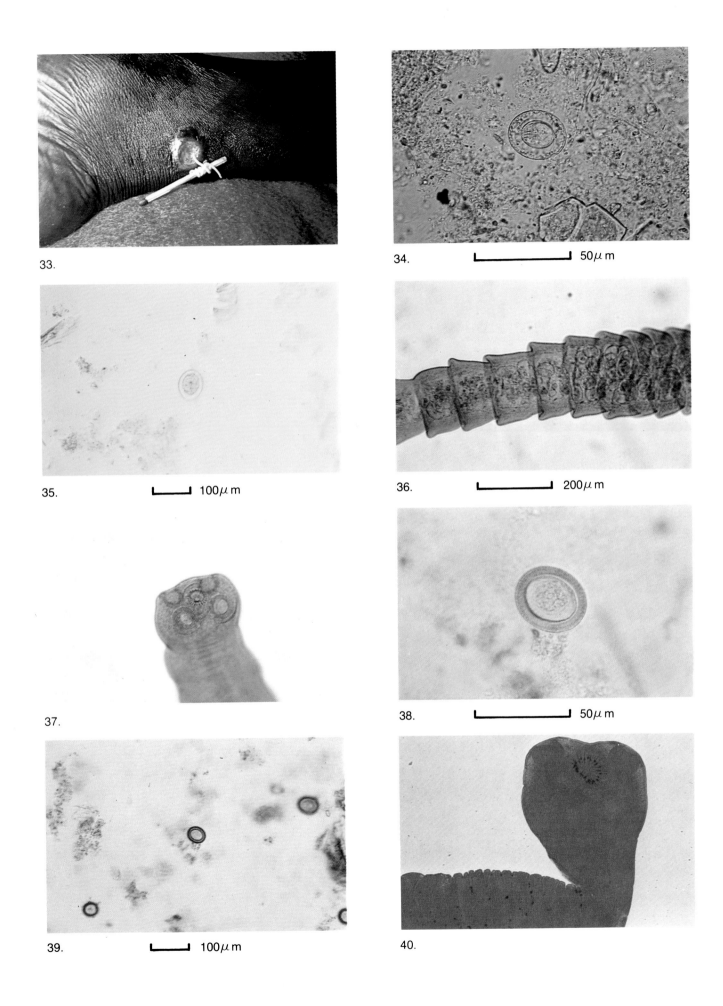

33.

34. |⎯⎯⎯⎯⎯⎯⎯| 50μm

35. |⎯⎯| 100μm

36. |⎯⎯⎯⎯| 200μm

37.

38. |⎯⎯⎯⎯⎯⎯⎯| 50μm

39. |⎯⎯| 100μm

40.

41. *Taenia saginata* (beef tapeworm) scolex (100×). This is the unarmed tapeworm; the scolex bears only four large, cup-shaped suckers and no hooks.

42. *Taenia solium* gravid proglottis (5×). The adult worm measures 2 to 8 meters in length, usually with fewer than 1000 proglottids. There are seven to thirteen (usually nine) lateral uterine branches (dark brown) filled with eggs in the gravid proglottis, which is diagnostic for the species when recovered in the feces. Gravid proglottids of *Taenia* species must burst open to release eggs because they have no uterine opening.

43. *Taenia saginata* (beef tapeworm) gravid proglottis (5×). The adult measures 5 to 10 meters in length and has 1000 to 2000 proglottids. There are 15 to 30 lateral uterine branches (dark brown) containing about 80,000 eggs in each gravid proglottis, which is diagnostic for the species when recovered in feces. The life cycle of both worms requires that the eggs be ingested by the appropriate intermediate host. The eggs hatch in the small intestine after ingestion by the intermediate host, and the six-hooked embryos penetrate the mucosal wall. They are carried by the circulation (blood and lymphatic) to various tissues where they encyst. Toxic metabolites and irritation at the site of attachment in the intestine by adult worms cause the human clinical symptoms. These are variable and frequently vague and include abdominal distress, weight loss, and neuropathies.

44. *Diphyllobothrium latum* (broad fish tapeworm) egg (400×). *D. latum* eggs (single size; 56 to 76 μm × 40 to 50 μm) are operculated (have a lid) and may be differentiated from operculated eggs of other helminths by the polar knob seen opposite the operculum, the size, and the undeveloped embryo seen within. Diagnosis is made when these eggs are recovered in stool specimens. Undeveloped eggs discharged from segments of the adult tapeworm must reach fresh water, where they mature and hatch, and the embryo infects the first intermediate host (copepods). Fish ingest infected copepods (water flea) and serve as the second intermediate host. Man acquires the infection by eating raw or undercooked parasitized fish containing the infective larval stage, the plerocercoid.

45. *Diphyllobothrium latum* egg (400×). The operculum of this egg is open. A polar knob is evident at the opposite end of the shell.

46. *Diphyllobothrium latum* egg (100×). A low-power view of the same egg.

47. *Diphyllobothrium latum* scolex (5×). The scolex of this species does not have hooks or cup-shaped suckers but is characterized by two grooved suckers, one on each side of the scolex. This worm attaches to the mucosa of the small intestine and can grow to 20 meters in length.

48. *Diphyllobothrium latum* proglottis (10×). The mature segment is much wider than tall and contains a rosette-shaped uterus. There is a uterine pore through which eggs are discharged. This parasite is found worldwide in areas around fresh water. In the United States, it is found in Florida, the Great Lakes region, and Alaska. The disease is often asymptomatic or is accompanied by vague digestive disturbances. Some patients develop a macrocytic anemia of the pernicious anemia type, because the worm successfully competes with the host for dietary vitamin B_{12} and absorbs it before it can enter the host's circulation.

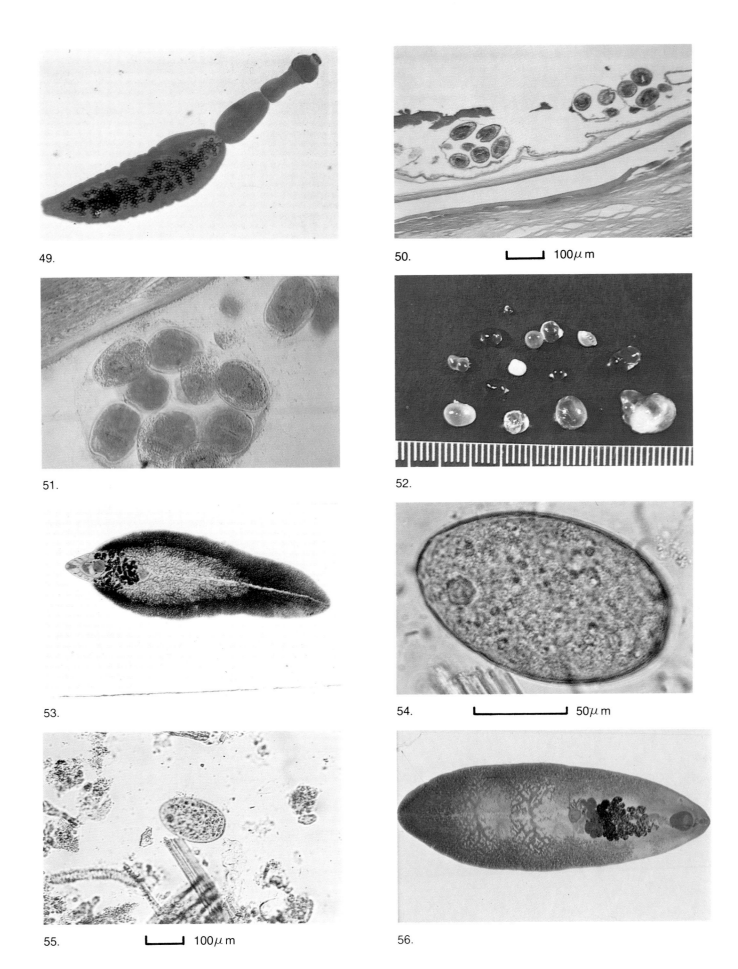

49.

50.   ⊢————⊣ 100μm

51.

52.

53.

54.   ⊢————⊣ 50μm

55.   ⊢————⊣ 100μm

56.

57. *Fasciolopsis buski* egg (400×). Recovery of this large, thin-shelled operculated egg (140 μm × 70 μm) is diagnostic. The operculum (lid) is visible here, open at the right end of the egg. This egg is empty; it was previously incubated, and the larva has hatched out of the shell.

58. *Fasciolopsis buski* egg (100×). Immediately below this large egg appears a *Trichuris trichiura* egg. These eggs give a graphic comparison of their relative sizes. The operculum is visible at the left end of the fluke egg, and the material inside is yolk. Most of the trematode eggs are undifferentiated when found in fecal specimens. Eggs of all species must reach fresh water before further development occurs. After full development occurs, the first larval form (miracidium) hatches and penetrates the soft tissues of an appropriate intermediate host, the snail. It develops through several stages to become a free-swimming cercaria which then encysts in fish or crabs or on aquatic vegetation as the metacercaria, which is infective if eaten by a human.

59. *Clonorchis sinensis* (Oriental liver fluke) (4×). This adult measures 1 to 2.5 cm × 3 to 5 mm. Man is infected by eating raw fish, the second intermediate host, containing encysted metacercariae. Larvae excyst in the small intestine and migrate to the bile ducts where they develop into adult worms. Visible structures include the oral sucker at the anterior end, the ventral sucker one quarter posteriorly to the oral sucker, the uterus (a dark branching structure extending downward from the ventral sucker to the ovary), and the testes immediately below the large, oval mehlis gland. The ceca extend from top to bottom toward the outer edge. The vitellaria are parallel to the uterus. This parasite is found throughout the Orient and causes obstructive liver damage with extensive biliary fibrosis. Symptoms result from local irritation and systemic toxemia. Loss of appetite, diarrhea, abdominal pain, and eosinophilia (5 to 40 percent) are common symptoms.

60. *Clonorchis sinensis* egg (500×). Eggs (15 μm × 30 μm) are deposited in the bile duct and are evacuated in feces. Diagnosis: recovery of this small egg in feces. Note the thick shell, the characteristic bell shape, and the thickened opercular rim (the shoulders). There is usually a polar knob opposite the operculum

61. *Clonorchis sinensis* egg (100×). A low-power view of a developed *C. sinensis* egg.

62. *Paragonimus westermani* (lung fluke) (4×). This adult measures 0.8 to 1.2 cm × 4 to 6 mm. Man is infected by eating raw crab or crayfish, the second intermediate host, containing encysted metacercariae. Larvae excyst in the small intestine; burrow through the mucosa; and migrate through the peritoneal cavity, the diaphragm, and the pleural cavity to the lungs where they develop into adult worms. Visible structures include the oral sucker at the anterior end, the ovary which is immediately below the ventral sucker about midway down in the organism, the dark staining uterus to the left of the ovary, and the testes located in the clear space beneath the ovary. The branching vitellaria are visible along the outer edges of the parasite. This parasite is found throughout the Orient, India, and parts of Africa. It causes a chronic tuberculosis-type disease with fibrous capsules forming around the adults. Eggs are coughed up in sputum which are visible as orange-brown flecks. Clinical signs resemble those of tuberculosis, including cough with bloody sputum. Adults may invade other organs. Symptoms vary with the location of the adult fluke.

63. *Paragonimus westermani* egg (300×). Diagnosis: recovery of this operculated egg (80 to 120 μm × 50 to 60 μm) in sputum or feces. Eggs can be found in fecal specimens when sputum is swallowed. Skin testing may provide better evidence of infections than fecal examinations. Notice the thin shell and the thickened rim around the operculum. There is also a shell thickening at the end opposite the operculum.

64. *Paragonimus westermani* egg (100×). A low-power view of the egg in the center of fecal debris.

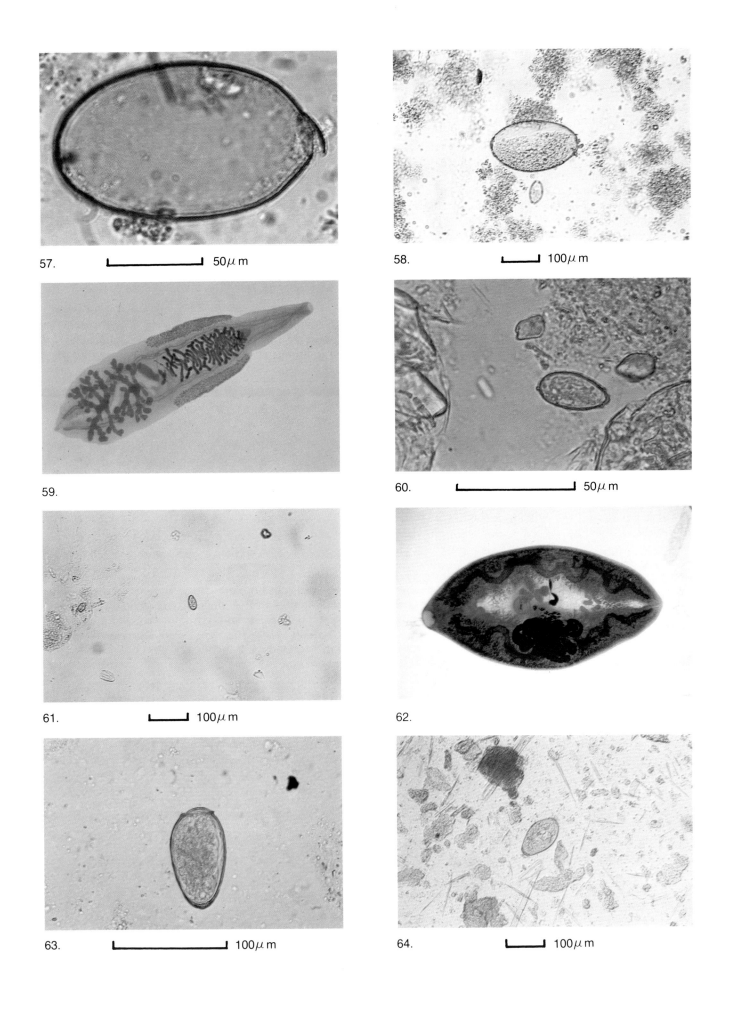

57.   50μm

58.   100μm

59.

60.   50μm

61.   100μm

62.

63.   100μm

64.   100μm

65. *Schistosoma* species (blood flukes). Adults are in copula. The female (15 to 30 mm × 0.2 mm) is seen inside the gynecophoral canal of the male. These unisexual worms have a cylindroidal shape and live in pairs, surviving for many years. Infection occurs when free-swimming, fork-tailed cercariae escape from the snail intermediate host, burrow into the capillary bed of feet, legs, or arms of humans, and are carried to the blood vessels of the liver, where they develop into adults. From there, *S. mansoni* and *S. japonicum* migrat to mesenteric veins around the colon. *S. haematobium* migrates to pelvic veins around the urinary bladder.

66. *Schistosoma mansoni* egg (400×). Diagnosis: recovery of eggs in feces. Unlike the other trematodes, schistosome eggs do not have an operculum. Note the large size (115 to 175 µm × 50 to 70 µm) and the conspicuous lateral spine protruding from the side near one pole. A ciliated miracidium is indistinct but visible inside this egg, but it is generally distinct and motile, with active cilia and flame cells in fresh specimens. Eggs are deposited into venules and eventually rupture the wall to effect passage into the lumen of the intestine and are evacuated in the feces. Many eggs are caught in tissues of the liver and intestine, and a granuloma forms around each egg in response to toxic enzymes released by the miracidium. Clinical manifestations include high eosinophilia (up to 50 percent), gastrointestinal bleeding, rectal polyps, and hepatic cirrhosis. This parasite is found in Africa, the Middle East, South America, and Puerto Rico.

67. *Schistosoma mansoni* egg (100×). A low-power view of several eggs. Note the lateral spines on the eggs.

68. *Schistosoma japonicum* egg (400×). Diagnosis: recovery of eggs in feces. This egg measures 70 to 100 µm × 50 to 60 µm. There is a small lateral spine on the egg shell which is characteristic for this species. A ciliated miracidium is seen inside the egg. The disease produced is similar to that of *S. mansoni*. Because *S. japonicum* produces ten times as many eggs as *S. mansoni*, the disease is more severe. Many eggs are swept back into the blood stream to the liver and trapped, causing fibrosis and cirrhosis of the liver. Toxic symptoms are severe. This parasite is found in the Orient.

69. *Schistosoma japonicum* eggs (100×). A low-power view of several eggs. The lateral spine is barely visible in some eggs.

70. *Schistosoma haematobium* egg (400×). Diagnosis: recovery of eggs in urine. This egg measures 115 to 175 µm × 40 to 70 µm. There is a pointed terminal spine which is characteristic for this species. A ciliated miracidium is visible inside. Egg deposition by *S. haematobium* causes local traumatic damage to the rectum and the urinary bladder. Bladder colic is a cardinal symptom. Blood, pus cells, and necrotic tissue debris are passed during urination. Systemic symptoms are less severe than those produced by the other schistosomes. There is a high correlation with bladder cancer in infected persons. This parasite is found in Africa, the Middle East, and Portugal.

71. *Schistosoma haematobium* egg (300×). A high-power view of the egg, showing a differently shaped terminal spine.

Amebae are unicellular protozoans, some of which may be parasitic in humans. These organisms are found worldwide, and some can live as parasitic or commensal trophozoites in the lower gastrointestinal tract of man. Most form a cyst stage (a dormant protective stage for the parasite in unfavorable environments after being evacuated in the host's feces), and in this form may remain viable for long periods in warm, moist conditions. Transmission of intestinal amebic diseases is from ingested cysts in fecally contaminated food, soil, or water. Cysts are most commonly passed by asymptomatic carriers.

72. *Entamoeba histolytica* trophozoite (10 to 60 µm) (1000×). This ameba is pathogenic for man. It can invade the intestinal mucosa, causing flask-shaped lesions and bloody diarrhea. It can also spread to other tissues, such as the liver, and cause amebic ulceration. Notice the nucleus which has a light chromatin ring at the edges surrounding a centrally located karyosome (compare with *E. coli*, Plate 78). The cytoplasm is finely granular as compared with that of *E. coli*. This is a trichrome-stained organism.

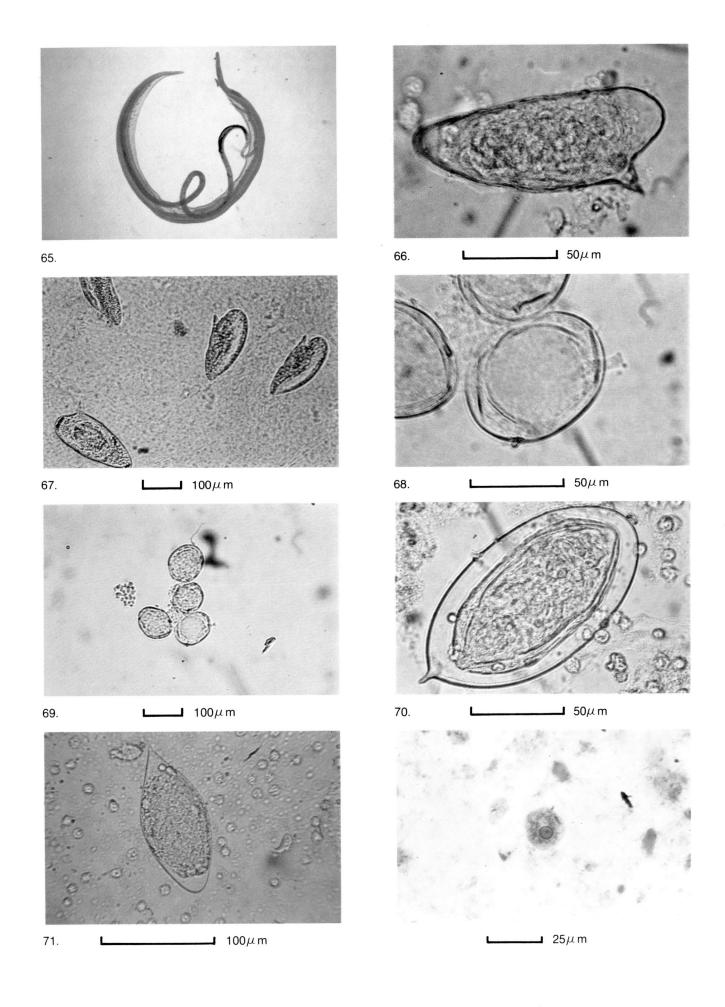

65.

66. |————————| 50μm

67. |——| 100μm

68. |————————| 50μm

69. |——| 100μm

70. |————————| 50μm

71. |————————| 100μm

|——| 25μm

73. *Entamoeba histolytica* (1000×). This trophozoite contains five engulfed red blood cells, the presence of which is a diagnostic feature, inasmuch as no other ameba will contain these.

74. *Entamoeba histolytica* cyst (1000×). Cysts of *E. histolytica* are over 10 μm in size (10 to 20 μm). There are up to four nuclei in the mature cyst. One nucleus is clearly visible here. The nuclear structure is identical in both trophozoites and cysts. The dark bars are chromatoid bodies which may be found in cysts. These are crystalline RNA. Iron hematoxylin stain.

75. *Entamoeba histolytica* cyst (1000×) showing four nuclei. Iodine stain.

76. *Entamoeba hartmanni* trophozoite (1000×). Note the morphologic similarity between the nucleus of this commensal and that in Plate 72. This organism was previously identified as *E. histolytica* but is now known as *E. hartmanni*. It is not pathogenic but morphologically resembles *E. histolytica*, differing only in size; it is less than 10 μm in size. This characteristic is important because correct diagnosis depends upon the careful measurement of the parasite. A trophozoite resembling *E. histolytica* that is less than 10 μm in diameter is classified as *E. hartmanni*.

77. *Entamoeba hartmanni* cyst (1000×). The cyst (5 to 10 μm) resembles that of *E. histolytica* but is classified as *E. hartmanni* because of its small size, the upper limit being 10 μm. This cyst is stained with iodine. It can have up to four nuclei.

78. *Entamoeba coli* trophozoite (1000×). This is a common commensal, and care must be taken to differentiate it from *E. histolytica*. Notice the nucleus, which has a dark, irregularly thickened chromatin ring around the membrane and a large, eccentrically located karyosome. This parasite is larger than *E. histolytica* (15 to 60 μm).

79. *Entamoeba coli* trophozoite (1000×). This trophozoite has a very large karyosome located next to the chromatin ring.

80. *Entamoeba coli* cyst (1000×). Five nuclei are visible in the cyst (10 to 30 μm). *E. coli* is differentiated from *E. histolytica* by the nuclear morphology and by the fact that the cyst contains up to eight nuclei, rather than four. Iodine stain.

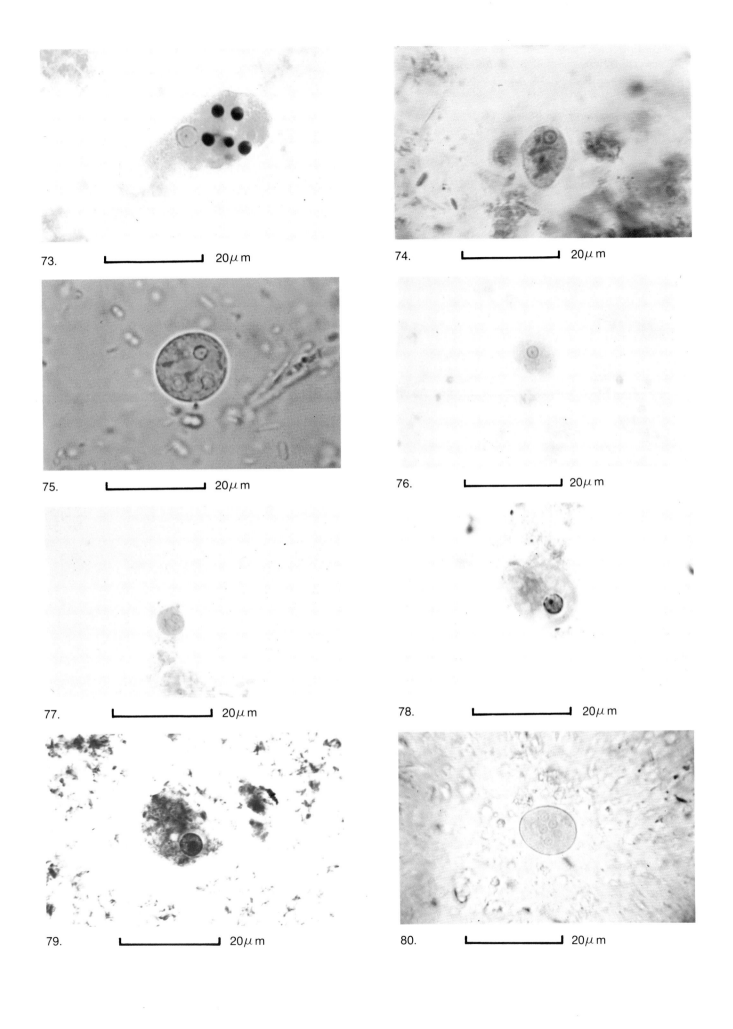

73.   20μm

74.   20μm

75.   20μm

76.   20μm

77.   20μm

78.   20μm

79.   20μm

80.   20μm

81. *Entamoeba coli* cysts (100×). A low-power view of several cysts. One is seen at the center of the field, and several others are evident in the lower left area of this view, all appearing as dark dots. This demonstrates the importance of scanning a part of all fecal slides under high power so that protozoa are not missed. These cysts also should be examined at higher magnifications in order to diagnose the parasite species correctly.

82. *Endolimax nana* trophozoite (1000×). Note the large karyosome in the nucleus. The fine chromatin ring is not usually visible. This feature is diagnostic for this commensal (6 to 12 μm). Note also the vacuoles.

83. *Endolimax nana* cyst (2000×). There are four nuclei in the ovoid mature cyst. Note the large karyosome (dark dots). The chromatin ring is not visible. These features are diagnostic. This parasite (8 to 10 μm) may be confused with *E. histolytica* if care is not taken when examining the nuclear structure and the cyst shape.

84. *Iodamoeba bütschlii* trophozoite (1000×). Note the large karyosome and light chromatin ring in the nucleus of the organism (12 to 15 μm). The cytoplasm is coarsely granular, and a small, light vacuole that contains glycogen is visible.

85. *Iodamoeba bütschlii* cyst (1000×). Note the large karyosome in the single nucleus of this trichrome-stained cyst (8 to 20 μm). A large vacuole from which glycogen has been removed by the staining process is visible (clear area inside cyst), which is diagnostic for this commensal. The glycogen vacuole will stain dark brown when an iodine wet mount is used. The nucleus does not stain with iodine.

Flagellates are unicellular organisms that move by means of flagella (motile fibrils extending from the body of the organism). Many of the flagellates have a trophozoite stage, which is the active, feeding, motile form, and also a cyst stage, which is a dormant, protective stage for the parasite in unfavorable environments outside the host's intestine. Transmission of the intestinal flagellates is by ingestion of fecally contaminated food or drink; *Trichomonas vaginalis* is directly transmitted during sexual intercourse; and the hemoflagellates (found in the blood or tissues) are transmitted by arthropod intermediate hosts.

86. *Dientamoeba fragilis* trophozoite (1000×). This flagellate (5 to 12 μm) does not form cysts. Note that there are two nuclei. This feature is diagnostic inasmuch as no other ameboid trophozoite has more than one nucleus. This organism may be pathogenic and may cause diarrhea in humans.

87. *Giardia lamblia* trophozoites (1000×). These flagellates (10 to 20 μm × 15 μm) live in the duodenum and generally do not produce disease. When present in large numbers, they may cause epigastric pain and diarrhea. Note the smiling-facelike appearance of the trophozoite, which is bilaterally symmetric with two anterior nuclei, a central axostyle, and four pairs of flagella. In fresh fecal wet-mount preparations, the motile trophozoite moves like a leaf falling from a tree.

88. *Giardia lamblia* cyst (1000×). Diagnosis: recovery of trophozoites or cysts (8 μm × 10 μm) in feces. There are four nuclei in the mature cyst, although there may be only two in the immature cyst. Three are visible in the upper cyst in this view.

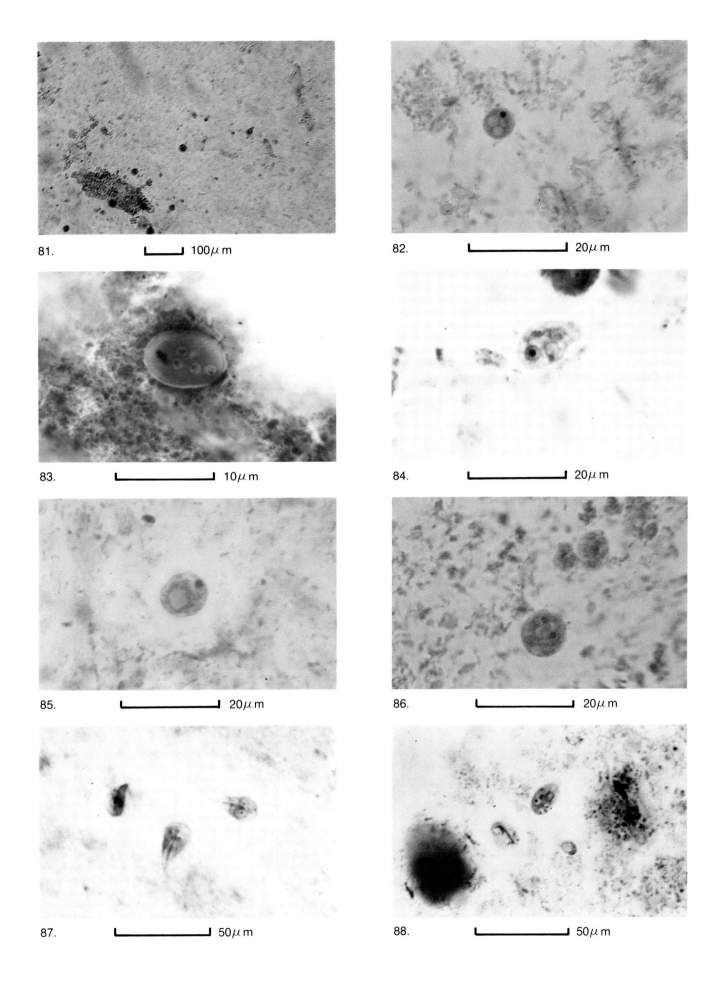

81. |———| 100μm

82. |———| 20μm

83. |———| 10μm

84. |———| 20μm

85. |———| 20μm

86. |———| 20μm

87. |———| 50μm

88. |———| 50μm

89. *Entamoeba coli* trophozoite containing several ingested *Giardia lamblia* cysts (1000×).

90. *Giardia lamblia* trophozoites (1000×). This stained section of duodenal mucosa shows two trophozoites adhering. Note the two nuclei visible in the trophozoite centered in the field.

91. *Chilomastix mesnili* trophozoite (1000×). This commensal flagellate (7 μm × 20 μm) lives in the upper large intestine and does not produce disease. Note the single prominent nucleus at the rounded anterior end. The posterior is tapered with a noticeably angled projection. There are four anterior flagella and a distinct longitudinal spiral groove. Viable trophozoites will move in a spiral path.

92. *Chilomastix mesnili* cyst (1000×). Diagnosis: recovery of cysts (5 μm × 8 μm) in feces. There is a single, large nucleus in this lemon-shaped cyst. Correct diagnosis is important so that this is not confused with *Giardia* or other pathogenic infection.

93. *Trichomonas vaginalis* trophozoite (1000×). This parasite (18 μm × 25 μm) is recovered in urine or in urethral or vaginal mucosal scrapings. Symptoms in women vary from mild irritation to painful itching, with a frothy, yellowish vaginal discharge. There are four anterior flagella, a large nucleus, and an undulating membrane (not visible in this view) extending along one half of the body. *T. vaginalis* appears slightly larger than leukocytes, and the whipping motion of the flagella is clearly visible in fresh, unstained fluid preparations such as urine. *Trichomonas* species do not form cysts. *T. hominis* is a nonpathogenic intestinal flagellate found in feces; *T. gingivalis* may be found in the mouth and is also nonpathogenic.

Two genera of flagellates are found as parasites of blood and tissue in humans. The *Leishmania* parasites have two forms in their life cycle: the amastigote form, which multiplies in macrophages in man, and the promastigote form found in the midgut of the sandfly, *Phlebotomus* spp. (the intermediate host). The second genus parasitic for man is *Trypanosoma*. These organisms take the trypomastigote form in the blood stream and other tissues in man, and the epimastigotes form in the arthropod intermediate host (except for *T. cruzi*, which also has a leishmanial form in man).

94. Amastigote form (1000×). Many amastigotes (3 μm to 5 μm in diameter) are seen in this view. The nucleus and the smaller, bar-shaped kinetoplast are visible in each organism as seen in the center of this field. The leishmania invade reticuloendothelial cells and macrophages of man. The disease produced by the organisms of each species is as follows:

1. *L. tropica* (Old World leishmaniasis). Local lesions occur at the site of the sandfly bite, followed by focal necrosis. Although it may be complicated by secondary bacterial infection, the disease is usually self-limiting and produces life-long immunity to reinfection. This parasite is found in Africa, India, and the Middle East.
2. *L. braziliensis* (New World leishmaniasis). The primary lesion is local, as with *L. tropica*, but the ulcer heals slowly. Erosion of soft tissues, especially of the nose, mouth, ears, and cheeks, often occurs years later, inasmuch as this organism tends to migrate to secondary sites, often complicated by bacterial invasion followed by local and systemic symptoms. This parasite is found in Central and South Americas.
3. *L. donovani* (kala-azar). The local primary lesion is usually not reported. The amastigotes gain access to the blood stream or lymphatics and eventually spread to fixed tissue macrophages. Sites of this invasion are the liver, spleen, and bone marrow, where multiplication usually proceeds unchecked. Anemia usually follows because of increased production of macrophages and decreased erythropoietic activity. The acute phase of the systemic disease is characterized by double spiking fever fluctuating daily (between 90° and 104°F). There is moderate erythrocytopenia, absolute monocytosis, and neutropenia. Massive hepatosplenomegaly occurs owing to parasite multiplication, and death frequently occurs if the patient is untreated. This parasite is widely distributed, except in the United States.

95. *Leishmania donovani* (1000×) seen multiplying in a macrophage in a press preparation of spleen tissue.

96. Leishmaniasis. A typical skin lesion caused by *L. braziliensis*. Note the open ulcer on the man's forehead.

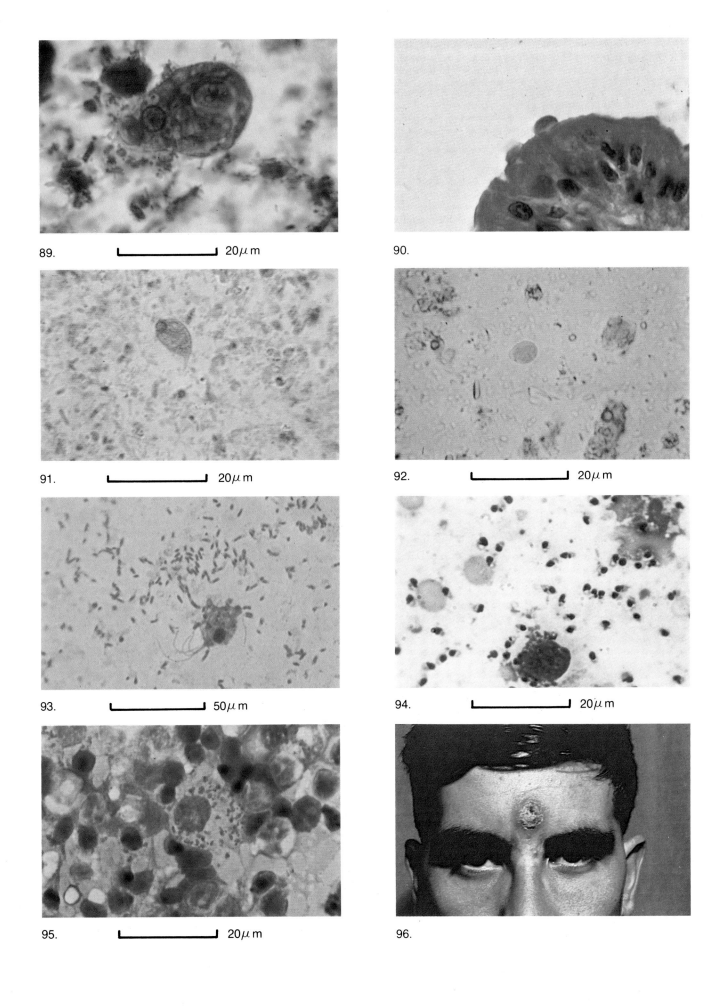

89. |⊢————————⊣| 20μm

90.

91. |⊢————————⊣| 20μm

92. |⊢————————⊣| 20μm

93. |⊢————————⊣| 50μm

94. |⊢————————⊣| 20μm

95. |⊢————————⊣| 20μm

96.

97. Promastigote form (100×). This stage is found in the midgut and later in the proboscis of the sandfly, *Phlebotomus*. It is the infective form of leishmaniasis and is transferred to man by the biting fly. The large nucleus, bar-shaped kinetoplast, and flagellum are visible. Note the relative position of these structures.

98. Trypomastigote form (1000×). The trypanosome is found extracellularly in the blood. It is the infective form transferred to man by the biting arthropod vector (intermediate host). Trypanosome species are not readily differentiated in peripheral blood. Visible structures include the flagellum, the large central nucleus, and the undulating membrane which is attached to the kinetoplast at the posterior end of the organism. The diseases produced by these organisms are as follows:

1. The sleeping sickness diseases produced by *T. rhodesiense* and *T. gambiense* are similar, differing primarily in the severity of the second stage, which is so severe with *T. rhodesiense* infections that death rapidly results. The disease begins with local inflammation at the site of the fly bite (tsetse fly). This subsides as the trypanosomes enter the blood. They migrate to the lymph nodes where severe inflammation occurs because of rapid multiplication. Toxic metabolites and occlusion of vascular sinuses by the proliferating organisms may cause death at this stage. Enlarged lymph nodes, myocarditis, fever episodes, edema, and rapid weight loss are cardinal symptoms for *T. rhodesiense*. Trypanosomes invade the central nervous system in the third stage to produce sleeping sickness and eventually death. *T. gambiense* usually proceeds to this stage. The posterior cervical lymph nodes in the neck are invaded and undergo massive swelling. This is called Winterbottom's sign. Other nodes may be invaded, producing weakness, pain, and cramps.
2. *T. cruzi* (Chagas' disease). The primary lesion at the bite site of the reduviid bug intermediate host is often near the eye, producing unilateral edema of the eyelid (Romaña's sign). Next, primary parasitemia with S- or C-shaped trypanosomes with a large kinetoplast occurs in the blood, causing fever and toxic conditions resembling typhoid fever (may be fatal in children). The chronic disease is characterized by leishmanial forms multiplying in tissue macrophages; and symptoms of tissue invasion, including enlargement of the spleen, occur; cardiac and central nervous system pathology occurs as tissue destruction continues. There may be fever episodes and parasitemia when trypanosomes are free in the blood.

Diagnosis of these diseases is confirmed when parasites are recovered in blood or seen in tissue specimens. Trypanosomes are 15 to 30 μm in length.

99. *Trypanosoma cruzi* (amastigote form) in cardiac tissue (1000×). The trypanosome in reduviid bug feces is pushed into the bite wound when the host scratches at the bite site, and these circulate in the blood until phagocytized, or they invade tissue macrophages, after which they change to the leishmania form. Note the nest of multiplying leishmania forms in the heart muscle.

The Ciliata

100. *Balantidium coli* trophozoite (400×). This organism (40 μm × 60 μm) is a ciliate which is characterized by having many short, ectoplasmic threads or cilia which are seen on the surface of both the trophozoite and encysted stages. *B. coli* is the only ciliate pathogenic for man. The disease is characterized by invasion of the intestinal submucosa with inflammation and ulcer formation. There may be fulminating diarrhea in heavy infections, or an asymptomatic carrier state in light infections. This organism has two nuclei: a large, kidney-bean-shaped macronucleus, and a small, round micronucleus (not visible in this organism).

101. *Balantidium coli* cyst (400×). This large, round cyst (50 μm) is characterized by the presence of macronuclei and micronuclei; the latter are rarely seen, but when present, generally appear as small dots near the concavity of the macronucleus. Cilia are evident around the inside edge of the cyst on the organism. This form, or the trophozoite, is diagnostic when recovered in feces or seen in intestinal tissue.

102. *Balantidium coli* cyst (100×). A low-power view of the cyst. This large parasite is easily recognized even at this magnification.

The sporozoa are protozoa that have both a sexual and an asexual phase in their life cycle. The genus *Plasmodium* includes the malaria parasites. The asexual phase is found in the human intermediate host, and the sexual phase occurs in the definitive host, the *Anopheles* mosquito. Sporozoites are injected into the blood by the biting mosquito and then invade liver cells. The asexual stages of malaria first multiply in the liver and later in peripheral blood. Asexual schizogony results in release of merozoites which either may invade new red blood cells and develop into new schizonts or develop to become male and female gametocytes. If the mosquito ingests gametocytes while feeding, these will develop throughout the sexual cycle to produce new sporozoites, the infective form for man. The clinical symptoms vary with the species of parasite, but all cause anemia (because of destruction of the red blood cells by the schizont form), headaches, general weakness, and a characteristic repetitive fever and chills syndrome.

103. *Plasmodium vivax* (benign tertian malaria). This drawing shows the erythrocytic stages of *P. vivax*. The prominent feature is the presence of Schüffner's dots. These appear as red spots on infected red blood cells on a stained blood smear and are seen in all developmental stages after the early trophozoite stage. The infected red blood cell is larger than normal red blood cells because the parasites preferentially invade reticulocytes, the larger, immature blood cell. The trophozoite divides to form a schizont containing 16 to 18 merozoites, which is a differentiating characteristic for *P. vivax*.

104. *Plasmodium vivax* (100×). A trophozoite is clearly visible in the center of the field. Note the red Schüffner's dots. Note also the ring (blue) and the chromatin dot (red). Each ring form (about one third of the cell diameter in size) represents one parasite; multiple parasites in a red cell are not commonly seen with this species.

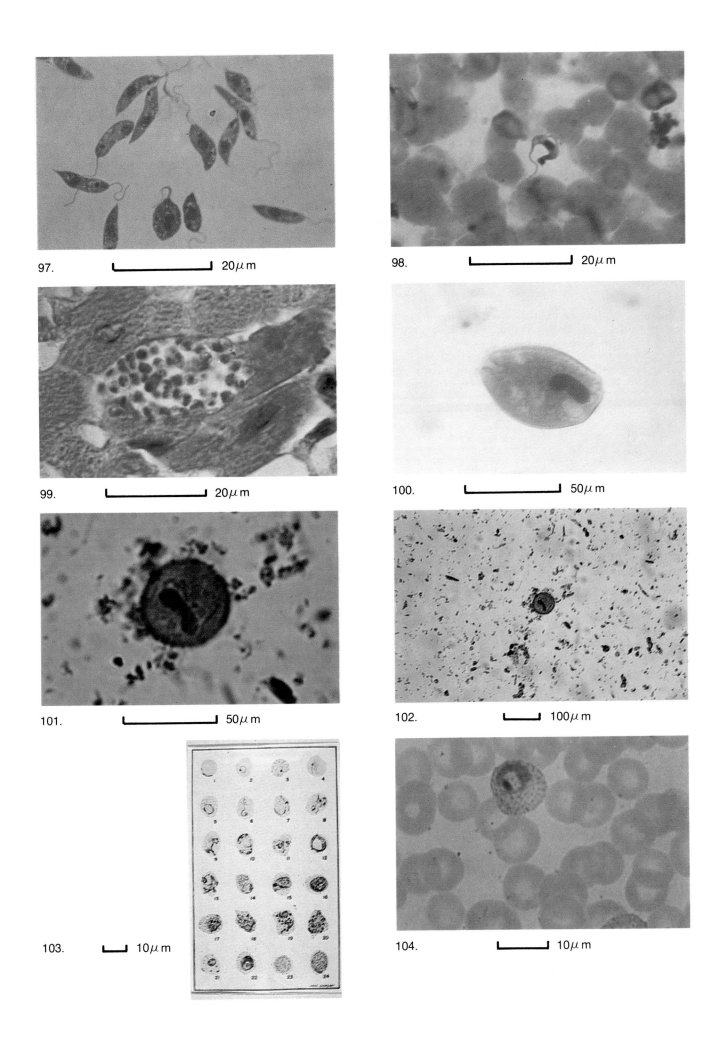

97. |⊢———————⊣| 20μm

98. |⊢———————⊣| 20μm

99. |⊢———————⊣| 20μm

100. |⊢———————⊣| 50μm

101. |⊢———————⊣| 50μm

102. |⊢——⊣| 100μm

103. |⊢⊣| 10μm

104. |⊢——⊣| 10μm

105. *Plasmodium vivax* (1000×). An older trophozoite than that in the previous plate is seen in the center of the field. Note the larger size of the red cell, the bizarre ameboid shape of the motile trophozoite, and the characteristic Schüffner's dots.

106. *Plasmodium vivax* (1000×). An older trophozoite than that in the previous plate is shown. This cell is enlarged and Schüffner's dots are evident. The trophozoite is clearly ameboid in its movements. Plates 104 to 109 clearly illustrate the maturation of the trophozoite stage of *P. vivax*.

107. *Plasmodium vivax* (1000×). Developing schizont. Many merozoites are seen inside the cell. A trophozoite appears in the lower left of the field.

108. *Plasmodium vivax* (1000×). Mature schizont. Fourteen merozoites are visible inside the cell. Characteristically, the schizont divides to form 16 to 18 merozoites. Development from the invasion of the red blood cell by the trophozoite to the fully mature schizont occurs in 48 hours.

109. *Plasmodium vivax* (1000×). Mature schizont. Eighteen merozoites are visible inside the cell. The red blood cell ruptures, releasing the merozoites which may invade new red blood cells to repeat the asexual erythrocytic cycle. Other merozoites may invade red cells and become gametocytes, which are part of the sexual cycle.

110. *Plasmodium ovale*. This view shows the erythrocytic stages of *P. ovale*. The red blood cells are enlarged and oval in shape. This parasite is rare in man and may be confused with *P. malariae* when Schüffner's dots are not present, or with *P. vivax* when Schüffner's dots are present.

111, 112. *Plasmodium ovale* trophozoites (1000×). This parasite is similar to *P. vivax* because Schüffner's dots are visible. It also resembles *P. malariae* because the mature schizont usually contains 8 to 12 merozoites. The diagnostic characteristic, when present, is the ragged, irregular appearance and oval shape of the red blood cell, as can be seen here.

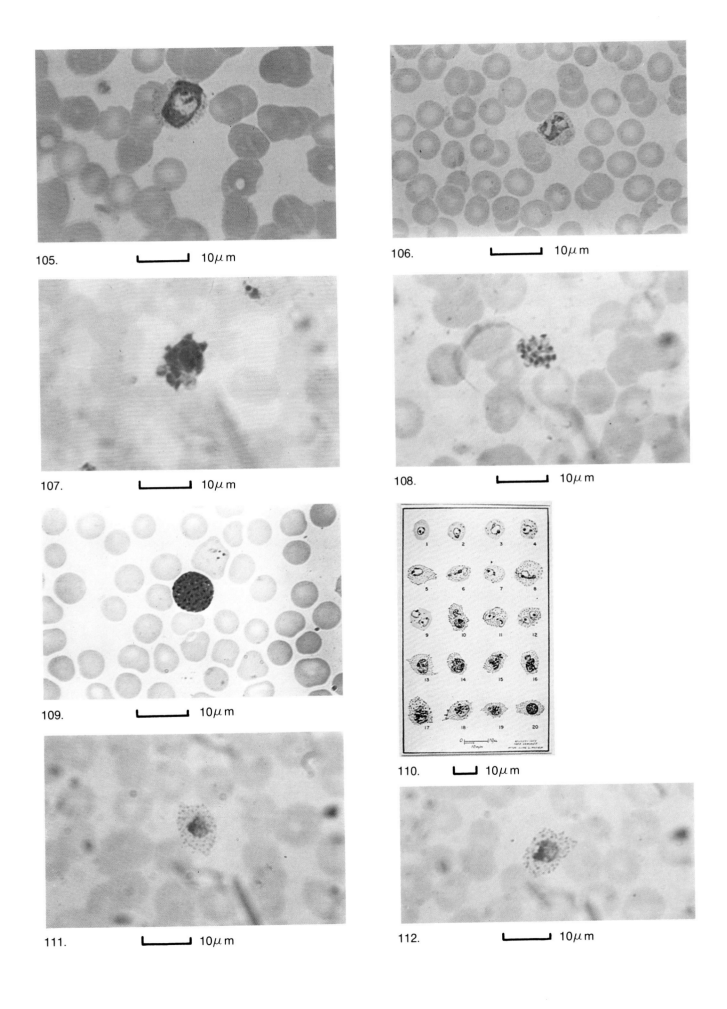

105.   ⊢━━━━┥ 10μm

106.   ⊢━━━━┥ 10μm

107.   ⊢━━━━┥ 10μm

108.   ⊢━━━━┥ 10μm

109.   ⊢━━━━┥ 10μm

110.   ⊢━┥ 10μm

111.   ⊢━━┥ 10μm

112.   ⊢━━┥ 10μm

113. *Plasmodium malariae* (quartan malaria). This view depicts erythrocytic stages of *P. malariae*. The tropho-zoite measures about one third of the diameter of the red blood cell. The prominent features include a large ring form; the band form of the early schizont with coarse, dark granules; and the mature schizont, containing 8 to 12 merozoites, which assumes a characteristic rosette shape with malaria pigment deposited in the center of the rosette.

114. *Plasmodium malariae* trophozoite (1000×). The band form trophozoite is characteristic during the early development of the schizont.

115. *Plasmodium malariae* schizont (1000×). A schizont containing seven merozoites is seen in the upper left corner. By 72 hours after the trophozoite entered the red blood cell, the mature form contains 8 to 10 merozo-ites and assumes the characteristic rosette shape. Two young trophozoites are also seen in this view.

116. *Plasmodium malariae* gametocyte (1000×). This form is similar to that of *P. vivax*, but is smaller and contains less pigment.

117. *Plasmodium falciparum* (malignant subtertian malaria). This demonstrates the erythrocytic stages of *P. fal-ciparum*. The prominent features are small ring forms with double chromatin dots, multiple rings in the same cell, and crescent-shaped gametocytes. Other stages in schizont formation are not seen in peripheral blood, because these (other) stages of maturation occur in the capillaries of internal organs.

118. *Plasmodium falciparum* ring forms (1000×). Note the small ring size and multiple infections, not seen with *P. vivax* or *P. malariae*.

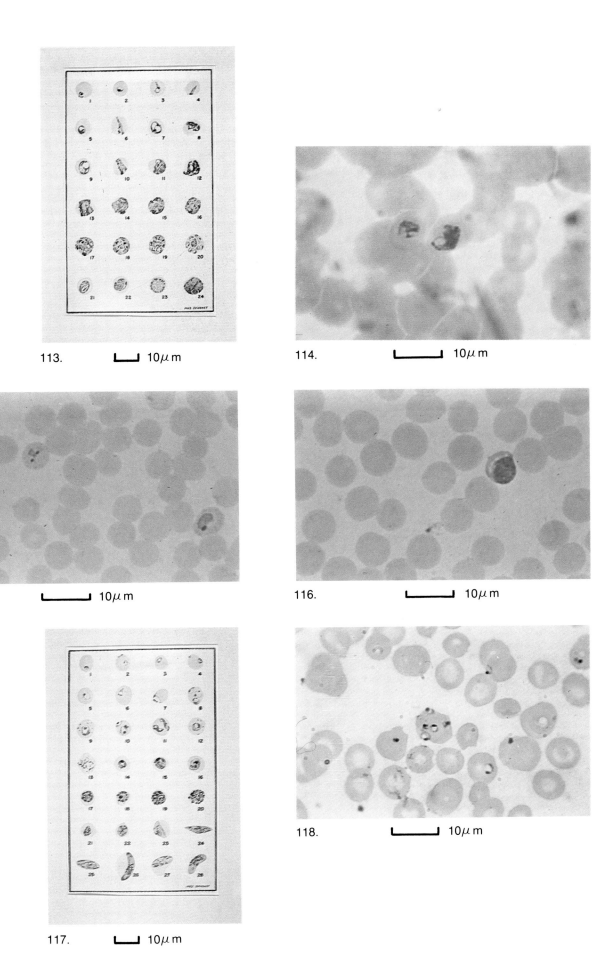

113. |⊢——⊣ 10μm

114. |⊢——⊣ 10μm

115. |⊢——⊣ 10μm

116. |⊢——⊣ 10μm

117. |⊢——⊣ 10μm

118. |⊢——⊣ 10μm

119. Double malaria infection (1000×). A *P. vivax* trophozoite is shown in the center of the field. The small ring form seen above it has a double chromatin dot, a diagnostic feature of *P. falciparum* rings.

120. *Plasmodium falciparum* gametocyte (1000×). Note the characteristic crescent or banana shape of this form.

Malaria has been found worldwide, but control measures have essentially eliminated the disease from many countries, including the United States. It is still a major problem in Africa, Asia, Central and South America, and the South Pacific. Diagnosis: clinical signs and observation of the parasite in thick and thin blood films obtained ideally during the fever cycle. Other important sporozoan parasites are noted below.

121. *Toxoplasma gondii* trophozoites (1000×). *T. gondii* trophozoites viewed by fluorescence microscopy in the indirect fluorescent antibody test (IFAT). This is a negative test result, indicating that patient's serum incubated with these organisms had no detectable antibody to *T. gondii*. No green fluorescence is observable.

122. *Toxoplasma gondii* trophozoites (1000×). This is a positive IFAT result for the detection of antibodies to *T. gondii* in serum. Note the green fluorescence over the entire body of the organisms.

123. *Toxoplasma* pseudocyst (400×). A dormant pseudocyst filled with bradyzoites of *T. gondii* as seen in a brain section. Immunosuppression of the host would allow these trophozoites to successfully invade new host cells and continue multiplication. These are also infective if ingested by the definitive host (cats) from mouse brains.

124. *Sarcocystis* spp. (1000×). A stained section of muscle tissue in which one can see a sarcocyst filled with potentially infective organisms. These are infected if ingested by the definitive host.

125. *Pneumocystis carinii* (1000×). A Romanovsky stained lung touch preparation. Note the cystlike structure in the center, which contains eight parasites.

126. *Pneumocystis carinii* (400×). A silver methenamine stain of lung tissue. Note the darkly stained cyst wall of the parasites within the honeycomb material in the alveolar spaces.

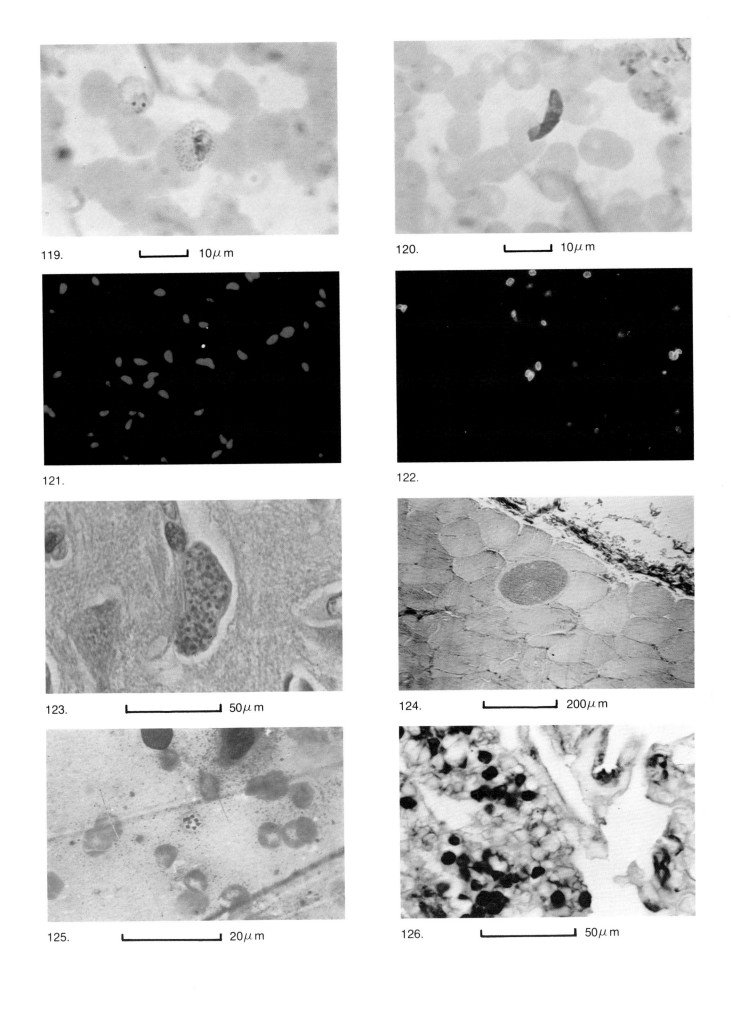

119. |——————| 10μm

120. |——————| 10μm

121.

122.

123. |——————| 50μm

124. |——————| 200μm

125. |——————| 20μm

126. |——————| 50μm

1

INTRODUCTION

North Americans do not suffer from a multitude of harmful parasites largely because of general good health; high standards of education, nutrition, and sanitation; a temperate climate; and the absence of certain appropriate **vectors.** Parasitic infections do exist in this country, however, and are still far from eradicated. Increased travel throughout the world and the general low level of understanding about parasitic infections have added to the problem of disease transmission in the United States. Many other parts of the world have levels of parasite-induced morbidity and mortality among humans and animals and parasitic damage to crops that are great drains on manpower and food productivity, thus affecting the international economy. In recognizing this problem, the World Health Organization named five parasitic diseases as among the six most harmful infective diseases afflicting mankind today.

To prepare you to identify organisms that parasitize humans, this book will explain parasitism as a biologic concept and will introduce specific parasites of medical importance, including the information necessary to assist in the diagnosis of infection. For substantive review of any particular parasite, you are referred to a variety of texts and specific journal articles in the bibliography of each chapter. Throughout the text you will find words in bold type (e.g., **vector**) which are defined in the glossary of each chapter; a medical dictionary, however, will be helpful to you in your studies. Pertinent references also have been included in the bibliography to guide you toward in-depth studies in various areas of parasitology, such as the biochemistry or immunology of parasitic infections. This text is best used in conjunction with a course that includes lecture and laboratory experiences. Treatment (drug or other treatment recommended) is also included for each organism infecting humans.

In order to function as a competent parasitologist, prepared to aid in accurate diagnosis of parasitic infections, you must exhibit knowledge and skills in both clinical and academic areas. This self-study text is designed to help you reach that goal. In addition to chapter presentations of each parasite, an extensive descriptive key accompanying the color photographs is located at the end of the book. These have been carefully chosen to provide a complete depiction of each parasite under discussion. The photographs and descriptive key are arranged in the same sequence as the species presented in the text.

The pre-test in this section is designed to allow you to evaluate your general knowledge of medical parasitology. Following each chapter, there is a brief post-test so that you may judge your mastery of that particular area. Learning objectives at the beginning of each chapter should guide your study. Review each chapter and plate key until you have completed your learning tasks as determined by a successful challenge of the post-test. A final examination at the end of the text will allow you to evaluate your self-paced learning accomplishment. A score of 80 percent correct must be achieved to demonstrate satisfactory completion of each chapter.

LEARNING OBJECTIVES

Academic Objectives. Upon completion of this self-study text, the student will be able to

1. state definitions for general terminology used in parasitology.
2. recall the scientific and common name for each parasite studied.
3. state the general geographic distribution of each parasite.
4. state the parasitic form that causes disease in humans and its body location.
5. describe the means by which each infection occurs.
6. state the name of the disease produced and its most common symptoms and pathology.
7. state the appropriate body specimen to examine for the diagnostic stage of each parasite and list other laboratory tests useful in its diagnosis.
8. recognize and draw the diagnostic stage of each parasite.
9. demonstrate graphically the life cycle of each parasite.
10. discuss the procedures used to identify parasites including concentration, culture, and staining techniques, as well as potential sources of error involved and quality-control procedures.
11. identify potentially successful methods for the epidemiologic control of parasitism.
12. given sufficient case history information, identify the most probable helminth or protozoan causing the symptoms and the body specimen of choice for study.

Practical Objectives. Upon completion of this self-study text and with appropriate experiences in the laboratory, the student will

1. be able to perform appropriate and satisfactory microscopic and macroscopic examination of body specimens—such as blood, urine, or feces—to detect and to identify parasites (acceptable performance will be the identification of 80 percent of the parasites present in specimens);
2. have mastered two fecal concentration techniques (one for sedimentation and one for flotation) as demonstrated by satisfactory performance of these techniques and correct identification of recovered parasites;
3. be able to prepare and to stain slides of fecal material and blood satisfactorily as demonstrated by the correct diagnosis of 80 percent of the parasites contained therein;
4. be able to perform a variety of other tests satisfactorily, including a fecal egg count; a blood concentration test for microfilariae; and serodiagnostic testing for various parasites.

PRE-TEST

The following questions will help you evaluate your general knowledge of parasitology. Allow 20 minutes for completion of the test. The multiple-choice questions are worth 6 points each; questions 11 and 12 are worth 20 points each. Write your answers on separate sheets of paper.

1. Pinworm disease may be diagnosed by which procedure?
    a. direct fecal smear
    b. cellophane tape test
    c. fecal concentration methods
    d. egg count technique
2. *Taenia solium* tapeworm infection occurs when
    a. undercooked beef is eaten
    b. eggs are ingested from contaminated soil
    c. larvae invade the skin of the feet
    d. undercooked pork is eaten

3. The most common helminth infection in the U.S. is
   a. *Necator americanus*
   b. *Ascaris lumbricoides*
   c. *Enterobius vermicularis*
   d. *Schistosoma mansoni*
4. The definitive host for *Plasmodium vivax* is a
   a. flea
   b. human
   c. mosquito
   d. fish
5. *Clonorchis sinensis* is commonly known as the
   a. beef tapeworm
   b. hookworm
   c. Chinese liver fluke
   d. bladder worm
6. The most pathogenic ameba in humans is
   a. *Entamoeba histolytica*
   b. *Entamoeba coli*
   c. *Giardia lamblia*
   d. *Balantidium coli*
7. Which of the following may be used to culture amebae in the laboratory?
   a. horse serum
   b. Wheatley trichrome
   c. loose moist soil
   d. Balamuth's medium
8. Xenodiagnosis is used for which parasite?
   a. *Schistosoma mansoni*
   b. *Trypanosoma cruzi*
   c. *Loa loa*
   d. *Wuchereria bancrofti*
9. Diptera is an order of insects including which of the following?
   a. mosquitoes
   b. lice
   c. fleas
   d. bugs
   e. ticks
10. The common name for *Necator americanus* is
    a. pinworm
    b. trichina worm
    c. hookworm
    d. fish tapeworm
11. Match the disease with the causative parasite:
    a. dwarf tapeworm disease
    b. threadworm disease
    c. traveler's diarrhea
    d. liver rot
    e. whipworm disease
    1. *Giardia lamblia*
    2. *Fasciola hepatica*
    3. *Hymenolepis nana*
    4. *Trichuris trichiura*
    5. *Strongyloides stercoralis*
12. Define or explain the following terms:
    a. vector
    b. host
    c. proglottid
    d. definitive host
    e. operculum

The answer key to all tests starts on page 171.

CLASSIFICATION OF PARASITES

I. Helminths—Metazoa; wormlike invertebrates. (Only those parasitic for humans are included in this text.) The following will be considered:
   A. Phylum Nemathelminthes
      1. Class Nematoda: roundworms (body round in cross-section)
   B. Phylum Platyhelminthes: flatworms
      1. Class Cestoda: tapeworms (body flattened and segmented)
      2. Class Digenea: trematodes, flukes (body flattened, leaf-shaped, and nonsegmented)

  II. **Protozoa***—unicellular eukaryotic microorganisms. The following will be considered:
  - A. Phylum Sarcomastigophora
    1. Class Lobosea: organisms that move by means of pseudopodia
    2. Class Zoomastigophorea: organisms that move by means of flagella
  - B. Phylum Ciliophora
    1. Class Kinetofragminophorea: organisms that move by means of cilia
  - C. Phylum Apicomplexa
    1. Class Sporozoa: organisms with both sexual and asexual reproductive cycles; **apical complex** seen with electron microscope.

  III. **Arthropods**—hard exoskeleton, jointed appendages. Only those that are parasitic to humans and those that transmit parasitic diseases will be considered.
  - A. Phylum Arthropoda
    1. Class Insecta: flies, mosquitoes, bugs, lice, fleas
    2. Class Arachnida: ticks, mites

GLOSSARY OF GENERAL TERMINOLOGY

Six glossaries appear in this text. In addition to the basic terms defined below, separate glossaries are included in the chapters on the Nematoda, Cestoda, Digenea, Protozoa, and Arthropoda.

Study and master all the words in each of the glossaries. It is recommended that the glossaries be used in conjunction with the bold-faced terms appearing in the text. A medical dictionary will also be helpful. Before taking each post-test, review the glossary included in the chapter.

accidental or incidental host. Infection of a host other than the normal host species. A parasite may or may not continue full development in an accidental host.

apical complex. Polar complex of secretory organelles in *Sporozoan* protozoa.

carrier. A host harboring a parasite but exhibiting no clinical signs or symptoms.

commensalism. The association of two different species of organisms in which one partner is benefited and the other is neither benefited nor injured.

definitive host. The host animal in which a parasite passes its adult existence and/or sexual reproductive phase.

differential diagnosis. The clinical comparison of different diseases that exhibit similar symptoms designed to determine from which the patient is suffering.

disease. A definite morbid process having a characteristic train of symptoms.

ectoparasite. A parasite established on or in the exterior surface of a host.

endoparasite. A parasite established within the body of its host.

epidemiology. A field of science dealing with the relationships of the various factors that determine the frequency and distribution of an infectious process or disease in a community.

facultative parasite. An organism capable of living an independent or a parasitic existence; not an obligatory parasite, but potentially parasitic.

generic name (or scientific name). The name given to an organism consisting of its appropriate genus and species title.

genus (pl. genera). A taxonomic category subordinate to family (and tribe) and superior to species, grouping those organisms that are alike in broad features but different in detail.

host. The species of animal or plant that harbors a parasite and provides some metabolic resources to the parasitic species.

in vitro. Observable in a test tube or other nonliving system.

in vivo. Within the living body.

---

*Classification derived from scheme adopted by Society of Protozoologists (from Cox, 1982).

infection. Invasion of the body by a pathogenic organism (except arthropods), with accompanying reaction of the host tissues to the presence of the parasite.

infestation. The establishment of arthropods upon or within a host (including insects, ticks, and mites).

intermediate host. The animal in which a parasite passes its larval stage or asexual reproduction phase.

Metazoa. A subkingdom of animals consisting of all multicellular animal organisms in which cells are differentiated to form tissue. Includes all animals except *Protozoa*.

obligatory parasite. A parasite that cannot live apart from its host.

parasitemia. The presence of parasites in the blood (e.g., malaria schizonts in red blood cells).

parasitism. The association of two different species of organisms in which the smaller species lives upon or within the other and has a metabolic dependence on the larger host species.

pathogenic. Production of tissue changes or disease.

pathogenicity. The ability to produce pathogenic changes.

reservoir host. An animal that harbors a species of parasite that is also parasitic for humans and from which a human may become infected.

serology. The study of antibody-antigen reactions *in vitro,* using host serum for study.

species (abbr. spp.). A taxonomic category subordinate to a genus. A species maintains its classification by not interbreeding with other species.

symbiosis. The association of two different species of organisms exhibiting metabolic dependence by their relationship.

vector. Any arthropod or other living carrier that transports a pathogenic microorganism from an infected to a noninfected host. A vector may transmit a disease passively (mechanical vector) or may be an essential host in the life cycle of the pathogenic organism (biologic vector).

BIBLIOGRAPHY

GENERAL REFERENCE TEXTS

BECK, JW AND DAVIES, JE: *Medical Parasitology,* ed 3. CV Mosby, St. Louis, 1981.

BELDING, DL: *Textbook of Parasitology,* ed 3. Appleton-Century-Crofts, New York, 1965.

BINFORD, CH AND CONNOR, DH: *Pathology of Tropical and Extraordinary Diseases,* Vols. 1 and 2. Armed Forces Institute of Pathology, Washington, DC, 1976.

BROWN, HW AND NEVA, FA: *Basic Clinical Parasitology,* ed 5. Appleton-Century-Crofts, New York, 1983.

CHENG, TC: *General Parasitology.* Academic Press, New York, 1973.

COX, FEG (ED): *Modern Parasitology.* Blackwell Scientific Publication, Oxford, 1982.

DAWS, B (ED): *Advances in Parasitology.* Academic Press, London and New York, volumes published annually since 1962.

FAUST, EC, BEAVER, PC, AND JUNG, RC: *Animal Agents and Vectors of Human Disease,* ed 4. Lea & Febiger, Philadelphia, 1975.

FAUST, EC, RUSSELL, PF, AND JUNG, RC: *Clinical Parasitology,* ed 8. Lea & Febiger, Philadelphia, 1970.

MARKELL, EK AND VOGE, M: *Medical Parasitology,* ed 5. WB Saunders, Philadelphia, 1981.

OLSEN, OW: *Animal Parasites.* University Park Press, Baltimore, 1974.

SCHMIDT, GD AND ROBERTS, LS: *Foundations of Parasitology.* CV Mosby, St. Louis, 1977.

SOULSBY, EJL (ED): *Immunity to Animal Parasites.* Academic Press, New York, 1972.

STRICKLAND, GT (ED): *Hunter's Tropical Medicine,* ed 6. WB Saunders, Philadelphia, 1984.

TAYLOR, AER AND BAKER, JR (EDS): *Methods of Cultivating Parasites in Vitro.* Academic Press, New York, 1981.

WALL, KW: *Immunoserology and parasitic diseases in the diagnosis of infectious diseases.* In FRIEDMAN, H, LINNA, TJ, AND PRIER, JE (EDS): *Immunoserology in the Diagnosis of Infectious Diseases.* University Park Press, Baltimore, 1979.

WARREN, KS AND PURCELL, EF (EDS): *The Current Status and Future of Parasitology.* Josiah Macy, Jr., Foundation, New York, 1981.

ZAMAN, V: *Atlas of Parasitology.* Lea & Febiger, Philadelphia, 1979.

2

NEMATODA

LEARNING OBJECTIVES

Upon completion of this chapter and the supplementary color plates as described, the student will be able to:

1. define terminology specific for **Nematoda.**
2. state the scientific and common name for all intestinal nematodes for which humans serve as the usual definitive host.
3. state the body specimen of choice to be used for examination for diagnosis of nematode infections.
4. state the geographic distribution and relative incidence of nematodes of medical importance.
5. describe the general morphology of an adult nematode.
6. describe the development of parasitic intestinal nematodes from egg through adult stages.
7. differentiate the adult parasitic intestinal Nematoda.
8. given an illustration or photograph or an actual specimen (if given adequate laboratory experience) identify the diagnostic stages of intestinal Nematoda.
9. differentiate microfilariae found in infected human blood.
10. discuss zoonotic nematode infections of humans and symptoms thereof.
11. classify and discuss methods by which the Nematoda infect humans: include the scientific name of any required intermediate host.
12. perform generic identification of parasitic infections by detecting, recognizing, and stating the scientific name of parasites present in biologic laboratory specimens (given appropriate laboratory experiences, as described in chapter 7).

Use these learning objectives as guides for your acquisition of knowledge. Assure yourself that you have indeed acquired the information necessary to do each task described before you attempt a chapter post-test.

The **Nematoda** include both free-living species that are metabolically independent and parasitic species that have a metabolic dependence on a host species in order to continue their life cycle. As a group, the nematodes are referred to as roundworms because they are round when viewed in cross-section. The different species vary in size from a few millimeters to over a meter in length. There are separate sexes, the male being generally smaller than the female. The male frequently has a curved or coiled posterior end with **copulatory spicules** and, in some species, a **bursa.** The adult anterior end may have oral hooks, teeth, or plates in the **buccal capsule,** for the purpose of attachment, and small body surface projections, known as setae or papillae, which are thought to be sensory in nature. Body development is fairly complex. The exterior resistant surface of the adult worm is called the **cuticle;** this is underlain with several muscle layers. The internal organ systems include a complex nerve cord, a well-developed digestive

DIAGRAM 2–1. An Example of a Life Cycle

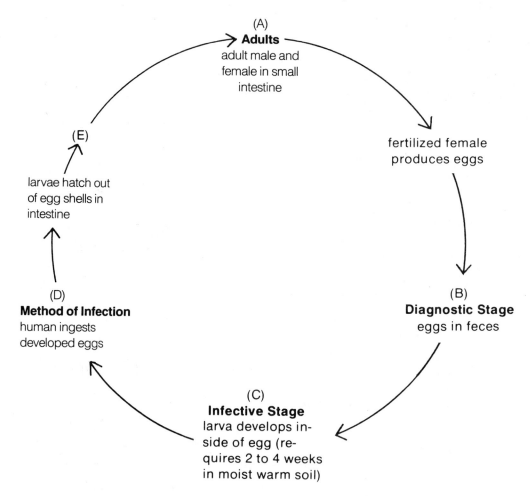

(A)
Adults
adult male and
female in small
intestine

fertilized female
produces eggs

(E)
larvae hatch out
of egg shells in
intestine

(B)
Diagnostic Stage
eggs in feces

(D)
Method of Infection
human ingests
developed eggs

(C)
Infective Stage
larva develops in-
side of egg (re-
quires 2 to 4 weeks
in moist warm soil)

system (buccal capsule, esophagus, gut, and anus), and complete reproductive organs are proportionally very large and complex. In the male, these include testes, vas deferens, seminal vesicle, and an ejaculatory duct. The female reproductive organs include ovaries, oviduct, seminal receptacle, uterus, and vagina. The female can produce from several hundred up to millions of offspring, depending upon the species. **Fecundity** is usually proportional to the complexity of the life cycle of the parasite.

Humans are the definitive host for the roundworms of medical importance, inasmuch as they harbor the reproducing adult roundworms. The adult female nematode produces fertilized eggs, or larvae, which may be infective to a new host by one of three routes: eggs may be immediately infective by being ingested; eggs or larvae may require a period of development to reach the infective stage; or eggs may be transmitted to a new host by an insect. Developing larvae generally go through a series of four **molts.** Most often it is the third stage larva (the **filariform** stage) which is infective. Infection of humans with roundworms can be by ingestion of the infective stage egg or larva, by larval penetration through the skin of the host, or via transmission of larvae by the bite of an insect.

The development of a parasite to the infective stage and the manner in which humans become infected are different for each parasite species.

Of the species of nematodes parasitic for man, about half reside as adult worms in the intestinal tract; the others are found as adults in various human tissues. The pathogenicity of intestinal nematodes may be due to migration of larvae through body tissues, piercing of the intestinal wall, bloodsucking activities of the worms, or allergic reactions to substances secreted by either adult worms or larval stages. Pathogenicity induced by the tissue roundworms is primarily due to immune and nonspecific host responses to the parasite secretions and excretions and to degenerating parasite material.

Depicted on the facing page is a generalized example of a **life cycle** which will show you the key points to study while learning about any parasite. Understanding the life cycle is the key to understanding how to break the cycle in nature, and thereby control the transmission of parasitic diseases. Minimally, the five parts noted on the diagram of the life cycle must be known.

A. Location of the parasite stage in a human host (e.g., adults in intestinal tract).
B. The means by which parasite stages leave the human host (e.g., eggs in feces). This is usually the parasite stage that is seen and identified in the laboratory. A parasite stage that is so recognized in any biologic specimen and thus serves as a key to diagnosis is termed the **diagnostic stage.**
C. The parasite stage that is infective to humans is termed the **infective stage.** It must be noted if external development is required for the parasite to reach infectivity (e.g., eggs develop in the soil).
D. The means by which a new human host is infected (e.g., egg is ingested).
E. Sites of development and maturation of the parasite in man.

GLOSSARY

NEMATODA. A class of the animal phylum Nemathelminthes—the roundworms.

buccal capsule (cavity). Oral cavity of roundworms. (In the case of hookworms, the cavity contains either cutting plates or cutting teeth.)

bursa (pl. **bursae**). Fan-shaped cartilage expansion at the posterior end of some male nematodes (e.g., hookworms).

copulatory spicules. Needlelike bodies possessed by some male nematodes; spicules lie in pouches near ejaculatory duct and may be inserted in the vagina of the female worm during copulation.

corticated. Possessing an outer mammillated, albuminous coating, as on the eggs of *Ascaris lumbricoides.*

cutaneous larval migrans. A disease caused by the migration of larvae of *Ancylostoma* spp. (dog or cat hookworm) or other helminth under the skin of humans. Larval migration is marked by thin, red, papular lines of eruption. Also termed creeping eruption.

cuticle. The surface of roundworms; a tough protective covering that is resistant to digestion.

dermatitis. Inflammation of the skin.

diagnostic stage. A developmental stage of a pathogenic organism that can be detected in human body secretions, discharges, feces, blood, or tissue by chemical means or microscopic observations as an aid in diagnosis.

diurnal. Occurring during the daytime.

edema. Unusual excess fluid in tissue, causing swelling.

elephantiasis. Overgrowth of the skin and subcutaneous tissue due to obstructed circulation in the lymphatic vessels; occurs in the presence of some long-term filaria infections (e.g., *Wuchereria bancrofti).*

embryonation. The development of a fertilized helminth embryo into a larva.

enteritis. Inflammation of the intestine.

fecundity. Reproductive capacity.

filaria (pl. **filariae**). A nematode worm of the order *Spirurida;* requires an arthropod intermediate host for transmission.

filariform larva. Infective, nonfeeding, sheathed, third-stage larva; long, slender esophagus.

gravid. Pregnant; female has developing eggs, embryos, or larvae in reproductive organs.

immunosuppression. Depressed immune response system; can accompany various diseases or be drug induced.

incubation period. The time from initial infection until the onset of clinical symptoms of a disease.

infective stage. The stage of a parasite at which it is capable of entering the host and continuing development within the host.

intermediate host. A species of animal that serves as host for only the larval or sexually immature stages of parasite development. Required part of the life cycle of that parasite.

larva (pl. larvae). An immature stage in the development of a worm before it becomes a mature adult. Nematodes **molt** several times during development, and each subsequent larval stage is increasingly mature.

life cycle. Entrance into a host, growth, development, reproduction, and transmission of a parasite to a new host.

microfilaria (pl. microfilariae). A term used for the embryo of a filaria, usually in the blood or tissue of humans; ingested by the arthropod intermediate host.

molt. A process of replacement of the old cuticle with an inner new one and subsequent shedding of the old outer cuticle to allow for the growth and development of the larva; the actual shedding of the old cuticle is termed ecdysis.

occult. Hidden; not apparent.

parthenogenic. Capable of unisexual reproduction; no fertilization is required, e.g., *Strongyloides stercoralis* parasitic female.

periodicity. Recurring at a regular time period.

prepatent period. The time elapsing between initial infection with the parasite and reproduction by the adult parasite.

pruritus. Intense itching.

rectal prolapse. Weakening of the rectal musculature resulting in a "falling down" of the rectum; occasionally seen in heavy whipworm infections, particularly in children.

rhabditiform larva. Noninfective, feeding, first-stage larva; has an hourglass-shaped esophagus.

tropical eosinophilia. A disease syndrome associated with high levels of blood eosinophils and an asthmalike syndrome. Caused by zoonotic filaria (or other nematode) infections in which there are usually no microfilariae detectable in peripheral blood.

visceral larval migrans. A disease in humans caused by the migration of the roundworm *Toxocara canis* or *T. cati* through the liver, lungs, or other organs. The normal host of these ascarids is the dog or cat. The disease is characterized by hypereosinophilia and hepatomegaly, and frequently by pneumonia. Migrating larvae can invade ocular spaces and cause retinal damage.

zoonosis (pl. zoonoses). A disease involving a parasite for which the normal host is an animal but which has accidentally infected a human.

INTESTINAL NEMATODES

In Table 2–1 you will find listed the scientific names (the genus and species names) and also the common names for the intestinal roundworms of medical importance that are included in this section. On the following pages are the life cycle diagrams, disease names, some of the major pathology and symptoms caused by infection with these roundworms, distribution, and other points of diagnostic importance. When you complete the study of these charts, you should be able to write

1. the scientific name
2. the common name

TABLE 2–1. Intestinal Roundworms

Order	Scientific Name (Genus and Species)	Common Name
Oxyurida	*Enterobius vermicularis* (en"tur-o'bee-us/vur-mick-yoo-lair'is)	pinworm, seatworm
Enoplida	*Trichuris trichiura* (trick-yoo'ris/trick"ee-yoo'ruh)	whipworm
Ascaridida	*Ascaris lumbricoides* (as'kar-is/lum-bri-koy'deez)	large intestinal roundworm
Strongylida	*Necator americanus* (ne-kay'tur/ah-merr"i-kay'nus)	New World hookworm
Strongylida	*Ancylostoma duodenale* (an"si-los'tuh-muh/dew"o-de-nay'lee)	Old World hookworm
Rhabditida	*Strongyloides stercoralis* (stron"ji-loy'-deez/stur"ko-ray'lis)	threadworm
Enoplida	*Trichinella spiralis* (trick"i-nel'uh/spy-ray'lis)	trichina worm

3. the location of the adults in humans
4. the diagnostic stage and body specimen of choice for examination
5. the method of infection of humans
6. other specific information pertinent to the diagnosis of each parasitic infection

Proper pronunciation of the scientific name is given beneath each name. Practice pronouncing the scientific name aloud and spelling it on paper.

In addition to the life cycle charts, Table 2–2 will help you review the pertinent information for each parasite, including the **epidemiology** and the major disease manifestations caused by these parasites. The second section of this chapter covers the tissue nematodes in the same manner as the intestinal nematodes, and the third section discusses zoonotic diseases. Be sure to study the corresponding pictures and descriptive key found in the color atlas at the front of the book while learning the text material. All other chapters of this book follow the same format.

When you feel you have mastered these materials (as outlined in the learning objectives), you are ready to take the post-test on the section. The directions for each test are included on the test pages, and the answer key begins on page 171.

DIAGRAM 2–2. *Enterobius vermicularis* (pinworm, seatworm)

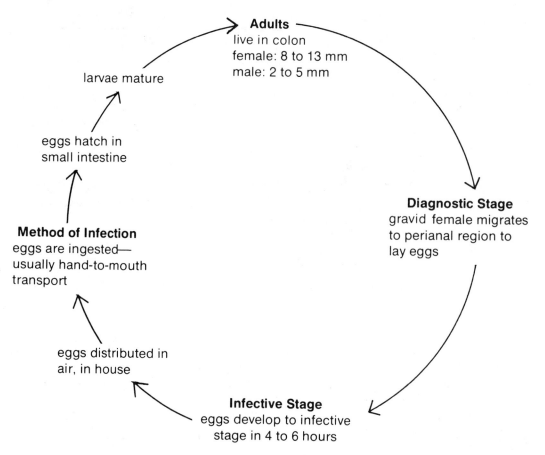

Adults
live in colon
female: 8 to 13 mm
male: 2 to 5 mm

larvae mature

eggs hatch in
small intestine

Method of Infection
eggs are ingested—
usually hand-to-mouth
transport

eggs distributed in
air, in house

Diagnostic Stage
gravid female migrates
to perianal region to
lay eggs

Infective Stage
eggs develop to infective
stage in 4 to 6 hours

METHOD OF DIAGNOSIS

Recover eggs or adult from perianal region with a cellophane tape preparation taken early in the morning when the patient first wakes. (See page 129.)

DIAGNOSTIC STAGE

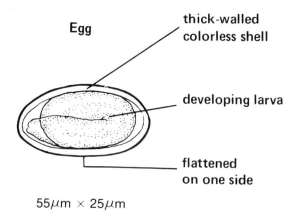

Egg

thick-walled
colorless shell

developing larva

flattened
on one side

55μm × 25μm

DISEASE NAMES

Enterobiasis, pinworm infection

MAJOR PATHOLOGY AND SYMPTOMS

1. At least one third of all cases are asymptomatic.
2. Rarely causes serious lesions; usually limited to minute ulcers and mild inflammation of intestine.
3. Other symptoms are associated with the migration of the **gravid** female out from the anus to lay her eggs on the perianal region at night.
   a. cardinal feature is hypersensitivity reaction causing severe perianal itching; eggs get on hands from scratching;
   b. mild nausea or vomiting;
   c. loss of sleep, irritability;
   d. slight irritation to intestinal mucosa;
   e. vulval irritation in girls from migrating worms.

TREATMENT

Mebendazole or pyrantel pamoate

DISTRIBUTION

Worldwide but more prevalent in temperate climates. Higher incidence in Caucasians than in Negroes. Most common helminth infection in the USA. It is a group infection, especially common among children.

OF NOTE

1. Humans are the only known host.
2. Each female produces up to 15,000 eggs. Most eggs remain infective for only a few days. Cleaning eggs from the environment and treating all persons in the household is important in order to break life cycle.
3. Eggs are rarely found in fecal samples because release is external to the intestine. Adult females can be occasionally recovered on tape preparation.

DIAGRAM 2–3. *Trichuris trichiura* (whipworm)

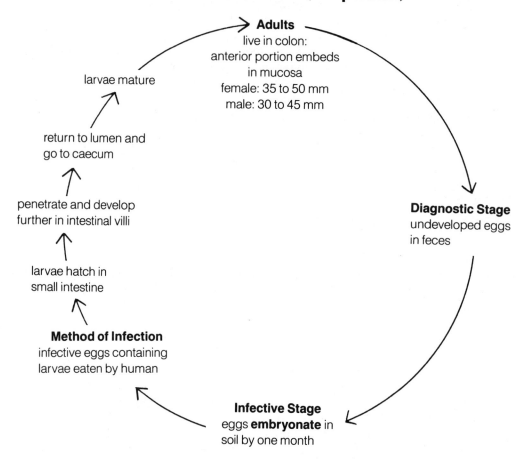

Adults
live in colon:
anterior portion embeds
in mucosa
female: 35 to 50 mm
male: 30 to 45 mm

larvae mature

return to lumen and
go to caecum

penetrate and develop
further in intestinal villi

larvae hatch in
small intestine

Method of Infection
infective eggs containing
larvae eaten by human

Diagnostic Stage
undeveloped eggs
in feces

Infective Stage
eggs **embryonate** in
soil by one month

METHOD OF DIAGNOSIS

Recovery and identification of characteristic eggs in feces.

DIAGNOSTIC STAGE

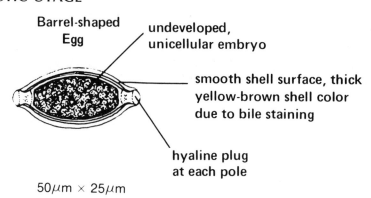

Barrel-shaped
Egg

undeveloped,
unicellular embryo

smooth shell surface, thick
yellow-brown shell color
due to bile staining

hyaline plug
at each pole

50μm × 25μm

DISEASE NAMES

Trichuriasis, whipworm infection

Major Pathology and Symptoms

1. Slight infection—asymptomatic. No treatment required.
2. Heavy infection—surface of colon matted with worms
   a. bloody or mucoid diarrhea;
   b. weight loss and weakness;
   c. abdominal pain and tenderness; colitis may be seriously debilitating;
   d. increased peristalsis and rectal prolapse, especially in children.

Treatment

Mebendazole

Distribution

Prevalent in warm countries and areas of poor sanitation. In the United States, prevalent in the warm, humid climate of the South. Third most common intestinal helminth. Common among children and institutionalized mentally retarded.

Of Note

1. Commonly, double infections occur with *Ascaris* because of the similar method of human infection.
2. Drug treatment may cause production of distorted eggs, which will have bizarre shapes when seen in a fecal specimen.

DIAGRAM 2–4. *Ascaris lumbricoides* (large intestinal roundworm)

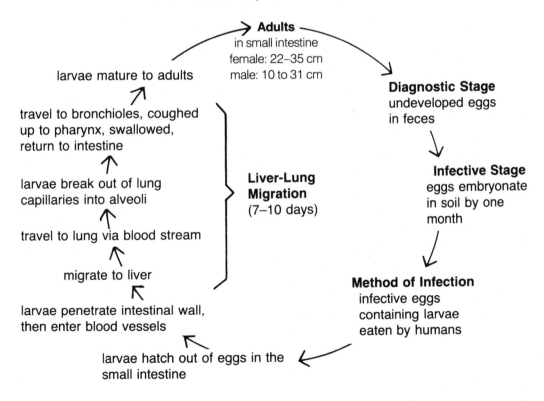

Method of Diagnosis

Recovery and identification of fertile (corticated or not) or infertile eggs in feces. Sedimentation concentration test recommended instead of flotation. Enzyme-linked immunosorbent assay (ELISA) serologic test available.

Diagnostic Stage

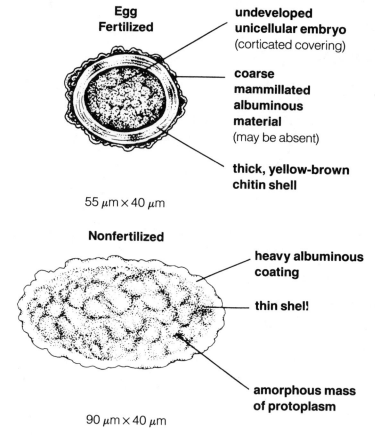

**Egg
Fertilized**

**undeveloped
unicellular embryo**
(corticated covering)

**coarse
mammillated
albuminous
material**
(may be absent)

**thick, yellow-brown
chitin shell**

55 μm × 40 μm

Nonfertilized

**heavy albuminous
coating**

thin shell

**amorphous mass
of protoplasm**

90 μm × 40 μm

Disease Names

Ascariasis, roundworm infection

Major Pathology and Symptoms

1. Pneumonia, cough, low-grade fever, and eosinophilia (Löfflers syndrome) due to migration of larvae through the lungs (1 to 2 weeks after ingestion of eggs). Allergic reaction may occur with reinfection.
2. Intestinal or appendix obstruction by adults in heavy infections.
3. Vomiting and abdominal pain due to adult migration.
4. Protein malnutrition in children with heavy infections and poor diets.
5. Some patients are asymptomatic.

Treatment

1. Mebendazole or pyrantel pamoate
2. Piperazine citrate

Distribution

Prevalent in warm countries and areas of poor sanitation. Coexists with *T. trichiura* in the United States; found predominantly in the Appalachian Mountains and adjacent regions to the east, south, and west. The eggs of these two species require the same soil conditions for development to the infective state, and infection for both is by ingestion of infective eggs.

OF NOTE

1. Ascaris is the largest adult intestinal nematode.
2. Adults are active migrators and may tangle and block intestine or migrate through intestine or appendix and out of the mouth or anus.
3. Ascaris is the second most common intestinal helminth infection in USA; the most common infection on a worldwide basis.
4. The adult female lays up to 200,000 eggs per day.
5. Eggs may remain infective in soil or water for years; resistant to chemicals.

DIAGRAM 2–5. *Necator americanus* (New World hookworm) and *Ancylostoma duodenale* (Old World hookworm)

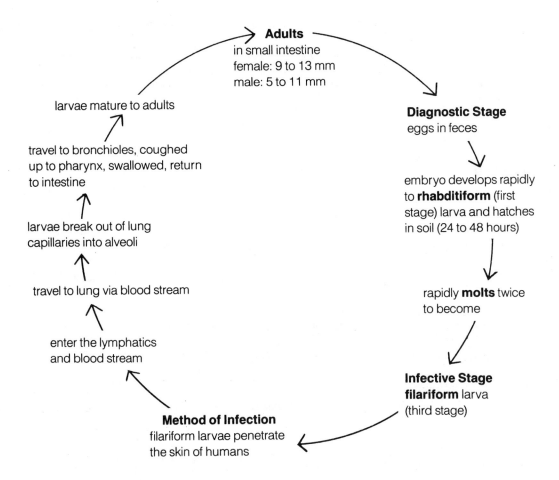

Adults
in small intestine
female: 9 to 13 mm
male: 5 to 11 mm

larvae mature to adults

travel to bronchioles, coughed
up to pharynx, swallowed, return
to intestine

larvae break out of lung
capillaries into alveoli

travel to lung via blood stream

enter the lymphatics
and blood stream

Method of Infection
filariform larvae penetrate
the skin of humans

Diagnostic Stage
eggs in feces

embryo develops rapidly
to **rhabditiform** (first
stage) larva and hatches
in soil (24 to 48 hours)

rapidly **molts** twice
to become

Infective Stage
filariform larva
(third stage)

METHOD OF DIAGNOSIS

Recovery and identification of hookworm eggs in fresh or preserved feces. Cannot differentiate species by egg appearance.

Diagnostic Stage

(*Note:* Eggs of these species are almost identical.)

Egg

thin, smooth colorless shell

two-, four-, or eight-cell stage of embryonic cleavage

50 μm × 30 μm

Disease Name

Hookworm disease

Major Pathology and Symptoms

1. After repeated infection, severe allergic itching at site of penetration of skin by infective larvae, known as ground itch.
2. Migration of larvae through lungs: intra-alveolar hemorrhage and mild pneumonia with cough, sore throat, bloody sputum, and headache in heavy infections.
3. Intestinal phase of infection:
   a. acute (heavy worm burden): **enteritis,** pain, microcytic hypochromic iron-deficiency anemia with accompanying weakness and loss of strength due to blood loss caused by adult worms;
   b. chronic (light worm burden): the usual form of this infection; slight anemia, weakness, or weight loss; nonspecific gastrointestinal symptoms.
   c. Symptoms secondary to the iron-deficiency anemia.

Treatment

Mebendazole or pyrantel pamoate

Distribution

Necator americanus—North America and Africa
Ancylostoma duodenale—Europe and South America
Other species in the Far East.
Common in agrarian areas.

Of Note

1. Moist warm regions and bare-skin contact with soil are optimal conditions for contracting heavy infections in areas of poor sanitation.
2. Delayed fecal examination can result in egg hatching and larval development; therefore, *Strongyloides* larvae must be differentiated from hookworm larvae (see color plates).
3. Heavy infection can result in 100 ml of blood loss per day; therefore, provide dietary and iron therapy support along with drug treatment as necessary.

DIAGRAM 2–6. *Strongyloides stercoralis* (threadworm)

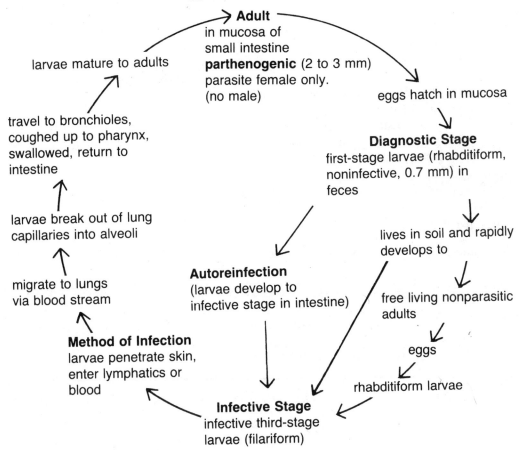

Adult
in mucosa of
small intestine
parthenogenic (2 to 3 mm)
parasite female only.
(no male)

larvae mature to adults

travel to bronchioles,
coughed up to pharynx,
swallowed, return to
intestine

larvae break out of lung
capillaries into alveoli

migrate to lungs
via blood stream

Method of Infection
larvae penetrate skin,
enter lymphatics or
blood

eggs hatch in mucosa

Diagnostic Stage
first-stage larvae (rhabditiform,
noninfective, 0.7 mm) in
feces

lives in soil and rapidly
develops to

free living nonparasitic
adults

eggs

rhabditiform larvae

Autoreinfection
(larvae develop to
infective stage in intestine)

Infective Stage
infective third-stage
larvae (filariform)

METHOD OF DIAGNOSIS

Recovery and identification of **rhabditiform** larvae in feces. Also, presence of hook-wormlike eggs in duodenal drainage fluid is diagnostic. (Larvae must be differentiated from hookworm larvae when found in feces; see color plate key.) Serology: ELISA.

DIAGNOSTIC STAGE

Rhabditiform larva
(*Note:* **Egg resembles hookworm egg.**)

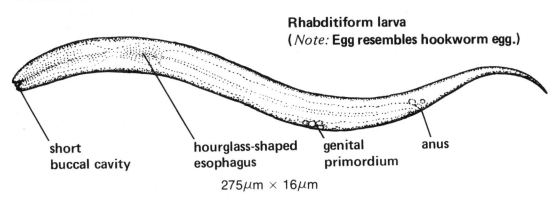

short
buccal cavity

hourglass-shaped
esophagus

genital
primordium

anus

275μm × 16μm

DISEASE NAMES

Strongyloidiasis, threadworm infection

MAJOR PATHOLOGY AND SYMPTOMS

1. Skin: allergic, raised itchy red blotches at the site of larval penetration upon repeated infection.
2. Migration of larvae: primary symptoms are in lungs; bronchial verminous pneumonia.
3. Intestine: abdominal pain, diarrhea and constipation, vomiting, weight loss, variable anemia, eosinophilia, protein-losing enteropathy. Frequently asymptomatic in light infection; gross lesions usually absent; bowel is edematous and congested in heavy infection.
4. Has caused death in immunosuppressed persons due to heavy autoinfection and larval migration throughout body, with bacterial infection secondary to larval spread and intestinal leakage.

TREATMENT

Thiabendazole

DISTRIBUTION

Warm areas, worldwide; similar to hookworm

OF NOTE

1. Parasitic female is **parthenogenic.**
2. Internal infection can continue for years because of maintenance of autoinfection.
3. Strongyloidiasis is difficult to treat.

DIAGRAM 2–7. *Trichinella spiralis* (trichinosis; trichinellosis)

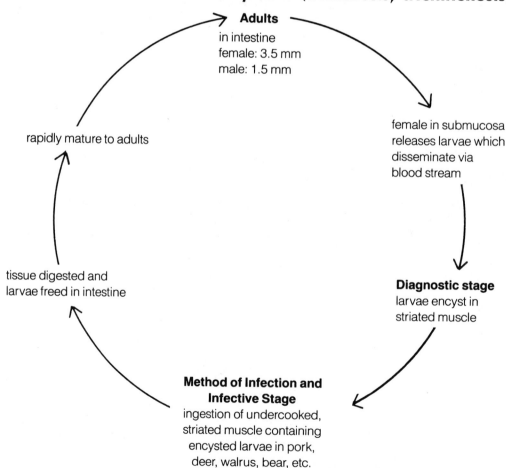

Adults
in intestine
female: 3.5 mm
male: 1.5 mm

female in submucosa releases larvae which disseminate via blood stream

Diagnostic stage
larvae encyst in striated muscle

Method of Infection and Infective Stage
ingestion of undercooked, striated muscle containing encysted larvae in pork, deer, walrus, bear, etc.

tissue digested and larvae freed in intestine

rapidly mature to adults

Method of Diagnosis

Identification of encysted larvae in biopsied muscle: serologic testing, three to four weeks following infection. A history of eating undercooked pork; with fever, muscle pain, bilateral periorbital edema, and rising eosinophilia warrants presumptive diagnosis.

Diagnostic Stage

Larva encysted in a muscle cell

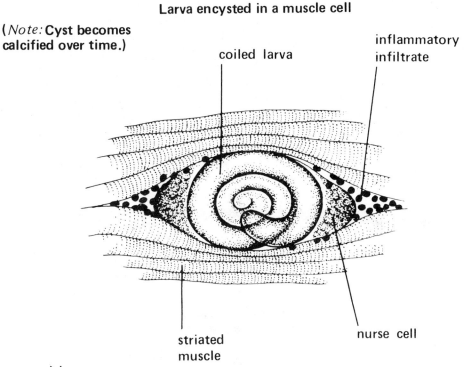

(*Note:* **Cyst becomes calcified over time.**)

coiled larva

inflammatory infiltrate

striated muscle

nurse cell

Disease Names

Trichinosis, trichinellosis

Major Pathology and Symptoms

1. Intestinal phase: small intestinal edema and inflammation; nausea, vomiting, abdominal pain, diarrhea, headache, and fever (first week after infection).
2. Migration phase: high fever (104°F), blurred vision, edema of the face and eyes, cough, pleural pains, eosinophilia (15 to 40 percent) lasting one month with heavy infection; death can occur during this phase in fourth to eighth week following infection.
3. Muscular phase: acute local inflammation with edema and pain of the musculature. Other symptoms variable, depending on the location and number of larvae present. Larvae encyst in skeletal muscles of limbs, diaphragm, and face, but invade other muscles as well.
4. Focal lesions: eyelid edema, splinter hemorrhages of fingernails, retinal hemorrhages, rash.

Distribution

Worldwide among meat-eating populations, rare in tropics. Prevalence in U.S.A. about 4 percent based on autopsy studies; only about 100 cases recognized and reported per year in U.S.A.

Treatment

1. Non-life-threatening infection (self-limiting): rest, analgesics, and antipyretics.
2. Life-threatening: prednisone. Thiabendazole (caution—effectiveness not proven, may have side effects.)

DIAGRAM 2–8. *Dracunculus medinensis* (guinea worm)

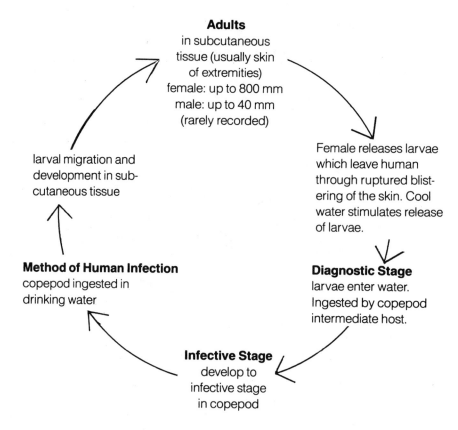

Adults
in subcutaneous
tissue (usually skin
of extremities)
female: up to 800 mm
male: up to 40 mm
(rarely recorded)

Female releases larvae
which leave human
through ruptured blist-
ering of the skin. Cool
water stimulates release
of larvae.

larval migration and
development in sub-
cutaneous tissue

Diagnostic Stage
larvae enter water.
Ingested by copepod
intermediate host.

Method of Human Infection
copepod ingested in
drinking water

Infective Stage
develop to
infective stage
in copepod

METHOD OF DIAGNOSIS

Visual observation of skin blister; induced release of larvae from skin ulcer when cold water is applied.

MAJOR PATHOLOGY AND SYMPTOMS

1. Allergic reaction during migration.
2. Papule developing into a blister which ruptures, usually on feet or legs.
3. Secondary bacterial infections or reaction to aberrant migration of larvae or adults may occur.

TREATMENT

Metronidazole, thiobendazole, remove adult from skin (slow withdrawal from blister or surgically remove).

DISTRIBUTION

Middle East and Africa

OF NOTE

Largest adult nematode

TABLE 2–2. Important Intestinal Nematode Infections

Scientific and Common Name	Epidemiology	Disease Producing Form and Its Location in Host	How Infection Occurs	Major Disease Manifestations, Diagnostic Stage, and Specimen of Choice
Enterobius vermicularis (pinworm)	Worldwide	Adult worms in colon; eggs on perianal region	Infective eggs are discharged by the gravid female on perianal skin; eggs are transferred from hand to mouth	Perianal itching caused by local irritation from scratching Diagnosis: eggs found by cellophane test (p. 129)
Trichuris trichiura (whipworm)	Worldwide, especially in moist, warm climate	Adult worms in colon	Ingestion of eggs containing mature larvae from infected soil or food	Light infection—asymptomatic Heavy infection—enteritis, diarrhea, rectal prolapse Diagnosis: eggs in feces
Ascaris lumbricoides (large intestinal roundworm)	Worldwide, especially in moist warm climate	Larval migration through liver and lungs Adult worms in small intestine	Ingestion of eggs containing mature larvae from infected soil or food	Light infection—asymptomatic Heavy infection—pneumonia from larval migration Diarrhea and bowel or appendix obstruction Diagnosis: eggs or adults in feces
Trichinella spiralis (trichina worm)	Worldwide	Adults in small intestine Larval migration; larvae encyst in striated muscle	Ingestion of encysted larva in undercooked meat (pork or bear)	Gastric distress, fever, eye edema, acute muscle pain, eosinophilia Diagnosis: encysted larvae in muscle biopsy; serology
Necator americanus (New World hookworm)	U.S., West Africa, Asia, and South Pacific	Larval migration; ground itch	Eggs shed in feces, mature in soil, larvae hatch and mature	Repeated infection results in larval dermatitis with later pulmonary symptoms

TABLE 2–2. *Continued*

Scientific and Common Name	Epidemiology	Disease Producing Form and Its Location in Host	How Infection Occurs	Major Disease Manifestations, Diagnostic Stage, and Specimen of Choice
Ancylostoma duodenale (Old World hookworm)	Europe, Brazil, Mediterranean area, and Asia	Adults in small intestine	Infective (filariform) larvae penetrate host skin, especially feet	Microcytic hypochromic anemia from chronic blood loss if heavy infection and poor diet Diagnosis: eggs in feces
Strongyloides stercoralis (threadworm)	Worldwide, warm areas	Larval migration; pulmonary signs Adults in small intestine	Immature (rhabditiform) larvae are shed in feces, mature in soil Infective (filariform) larvae penetrate host skin, especially feet Autoinfection by mature larvae in intestine Soil dwelling, nonparasitic adults may produce additional infective stage larvae	Repeated infection results in larval dermatitis with later pulmonary symptoms Heavy infections—abdominal pain, vomiting, and diarrhea Moderate eosinophilia Immunosuppressed host may suffer severe symptoms or death from heavy worm burdens inasmuch as autoinfection may occur Diagnosis: rhabditiform larvae in feces
Dracunculus medinensis (Guinea worm)	Africa, Asia, South America No periodicity *Cyclops* (crustacean)	Adults live in subcutaneous tissues; females migrate (Larvae released from skin ulcer)	Ingestion of water containing crustaceans infected with larvae	Systemic allergic symptoms and local ulcer formation Diagnosis: adult in skin ulcer, larvae released into water

Proceed now to study Color Plates 1 to 27.

FILARIAE

Table 2-3 gives the scientific and common names for the members of the superfamily *Filarioidea* (the tissue roundworms) to be discussed in this section.

TABLE 2–3. Filariae

Scientific Name	Common Name
Wuchereria bancrofti (wooch-ur-eer'ee-uh/ban-krof'tye)	Bancroft's filaria
Brugia malayi (broog'ee-uh/may-lay eye)	Malayan filaria
Loa loa (lo'uh/lo'uh)	eyeworm
Onchocerca volvulus (onk'o-sur'kuh/vol'vew-lus)	blinding filaria

GENERAL LIFE CYCLE

Adult filariae live in various human tissue locations. In general, fertilized adult female filariae living in the tissues produce living embryos (**microfilariae**), which migrate into lymphatics, blood, or skin. All these parasites require an arthropod **intermediate host** for transmission of infection. If the arthropod ingests microfilariae while taking a blood meal, they will molt twice inside the arthropod intermediate host and become the infective stage filariform larvae. These larvae are released from the insect's proboscis and enter a new human definitive host when the arthropod next feeds on blood. The entering larvae migrate to the appropriate tissue site and develop to become adults. Maturation can take up to a year.

In some species, the microfilariae are more prevalent in peripheral blood at specific times of the day (that is, exhibit **periodicity**). These times appear to coincide with the usual feeding pattern of the arthropod intermediate host species. Nocturnal or **diurnal** periodicity is noted in Table 2–4.

At least three other species of filariae are common parasites of humans. *Dipetalonema perstans*, found in Africa and Central and South Americas, and *Mansonella ozzardi*, found in Central and South Americas, apparently do not induce pathology but do produce microfilariae in the blood. *Dipetalonema streptocerca*, found in tropical Africa, produces microfilariae that are found in the skin, as does *Onchocerca volvulus*. Microfilariae must, therefore, be speciated, and these diagnostic stages are illustrated below to aid in differential diagnosis of filariasis.

Information listed on the following pages is keyed by number according to genus and species: **1** = *Wuchereria bancrofti*; **2** = *Brugia malayi*; **3** = *Loa loa*; **4** = *Onchocerca volvulus*.

DIAGRAM 2–9. Filariae

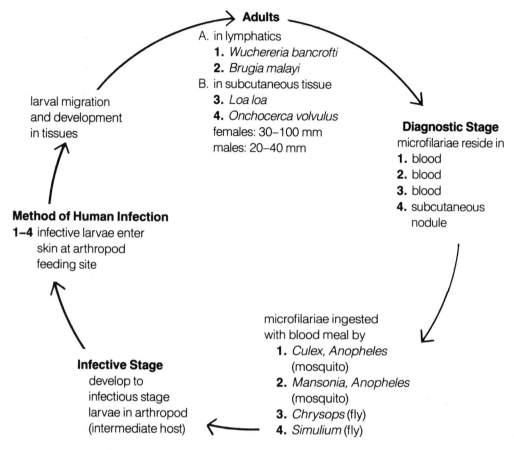

Adults
A. in lymphatics
  1. *Wuchereria bancrofti*
  2. *Brugia malayi*
B. in subcutaneous tissue
  3. *Loa loa*
  4. *Onchocerca volvulus*
  females: 30–100 mm
  males: 20–40 mm

larval migration
and development
in tissues

Diagnostic Stage
microfilariae reside in
  1. blood
  2. blood
  3. blood
  4. subcutaneous
      nodule

Method of Human Infection
1–4 infective larvae enter
  skin at arthropod
  feeding site

microfilariae ingested
with blood meal by
  1. *Culex, Anopheles*
      (mosquito)
  2. *Mansonia, Anopheles*
      (mosquito)
  3. *Chrysops* (fly)
  4. *Simulium* (fly)

Infective Stage
  develop to
  infectious stage
  larvae in arthropod
  (intermediate host)

METHOD OF DIAGNOSIS

A. 1–3. microfilariae (200 to 300 μm) in stained blood smear (see page 134). Also, can centrifuge blood sample and lyse red blood cells to concentrate microfilariae in the specimen before staining. (See page 135, Knott's technique.) 4. microfilariae in tissue scraping of nodule.

B. Serology (lacks specificity).

Differentiation of Microfilariae as Seen in a Stained Blood Smear

Examine for the presence or absence of a sheath (a thin, translucent eggshell remnant covering the body of the microfilaria and extending past the head and tail).

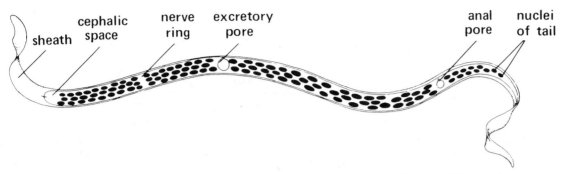

Examine tail area of microfilaria for presence or absence of cells that exhibit a characteristic array of stained nuclei.

A. No nuclei in tail

(1) *Wuchereria bancrofti*
sheath present

(2) *Mansonella ozzardi* **(nonpathogen)**
no sheath

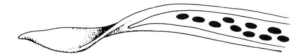
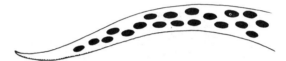
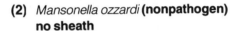

Tail of microfilaria of *Onchocerca volvulus* as seen in a tissue scraping from the nodular mass containing the adult filaria or from a skin snip (no sheath; nuclei not terminal, tail straight).

Tail of *Dipetalonema streptocerca* is bent like a fishhook. These microfilariae are not found in blood smears, only in tissue scrapings.

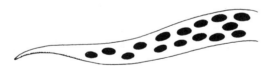

B. Nuclei in tail

(1) *Loa loa*
continuous row of posterior nuclei;
sheath present

(2) *Brugia malayi*
nuclei not continuous, two at
tip of tail; sheath present

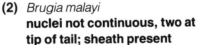

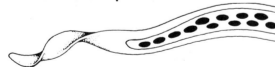
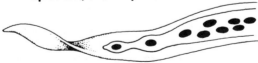

(3) *Dipetalonema perstans* **(nonpathogen)**
nuclei in tip of tail; no sheath

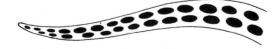

DISEASE NAME

Filariasis

1. elephantiasis, Bancroft's filariasis
2. Malayan filariasis
3. eyeworm
4. blinding filaria; river blindness

MAJOR PATHOLOGY AND SYMPTOMS

1–2. Early acute phase causes fever and lymphangitis; eventual chronic elephantiasis develops due to obstruction of lymphatics after years of repeated exposure. Adults in lymphatics sequentially induce dilation, inflammation, granulomatous thickening of lymphatic walls, and finally obstruction. Malayan filariasis is more often asymptomatic.

3. Localized subcutaneous edema (Calabar swellings), particularly around eye, because of microfilaria migration and death in capillaries. Living adults cause no inflammation; dying adults induce granulomatous reaction.

4. Fibrotic nodules encapsulating adults (Onchocercomas). Progressively severe allergic onchodermatitis (pigmented rash); blindness occurs from microfilariae in all ocular structures (very prevalent in Africa) and Central America (on coffee plantations).

TREATMENT

1. Diethylcarbamazine
2. Diethylcarbamazine
3. Diethylcarbamazine
4. Ivermectin

DISTRIBUTION

1. Spotty worldwide, tropical and subtropical
2. Far East
3. Africa
4. Central America and Africa

OF NOTE

1. Mosquito's resistance to insecticides and increasing coastal-dwelling human populations are increasing the incidence of exposure.
2. Eosinophilic lung (tropical eosinophilia), an asthmalike syndrome, may be caused by **occult** filariasis.
3. Onchocerciasis is the major cause of blindness in Africa; control is difficult because *Simulium* breed in running water.

TABLE 2–4. Important Filarial Infections

Scientific and Common Name	Epidemiology, Periodicity, and Intermediate Host	Disease Producing Form and Its Location in Host	How Infection Occurs	Major Disease Manifestations, Diagnostic Stage, and Specimen of Choice
Wuchereria bancrofti (Bancroft's filaria)	Tropics. Nocturnal periodicity.	Adults live in the lymphatics (Microfilariae in blood)	Filariform larvae enter through bite wound into the blood	Invades lymphatics and causes granulomatous lesions, chills,

TABLE 2–4. *Continued*

Scientific and Common Name	Epidemiology, Periodicity, and Intermediate Host	Disease Producing Form and Its Location in Host	How Infection Occurs	Major Disease Manifestations, Diagnostic Stage, and Specimen of Choice
	Culex, Aedes, and *Anopheles* mosquitoes		when the mosquito bites a human to take a blood meal	fever, eosinophilia, and eventual elephantiasis Diagnosis: microfilariae in blood; serology
Brugia malayi (Malayan filaria)	Far East. Nocturnal periodicity. *Anopheles* and *Mansonia* mosquitoes	As above	As above	As above
Loa loa (eyeworm)	Africa. Diurnal periodicity. *Chrysops* fly	Adults migrate throughout the subcutaneous tissues (microfilariae in blood)	As above, except the vector is a blood-sucking fly	Chronic and benign disease Diagnosis: microfilariae in blood; serology; Calabar swelling (a transient subcutaneous swelling)
Onchocerca volvulus (blinding filaria)	Central America and Africa No periodicity *Simulium* (black fly)	Adults live in fibrotic nodules (microfilariae migrate subcutaneously)	As above, except the vector is a blood-sucking fly	Chronic and nonfatal Allergy to microfilariae causes local symptoms— may cause blindness Diagnosis: adults in excised nodules; microfilariae in tissue scraping of nodule

Proceed now to study Color Plates 28 to 33.

ZOONOSES

Zoonoses are parasitic infections in which humans are accidentally infected with parasites that usually live in animals. Table 2–5 lists the scientific names of the parasites, their geographic locations, their normal animal hosts, and the disease and symptoms

TABLE 2–5. Important Zoonotic Infections

Scientific and Common Name	Geographic Location	Normal Animal Host	Disease	Symptoms in Humans	Method of Infection of Humans
Ancylostoma braziliense *Ancylostoma caninum* (dog hookworms)	Southern U.S., Central and South America, Africa, Asia, Northern Hemisphere	Dog Dog	Cutaneous larval migrans (CLM); Creeping eruption	Allergic response to the migration of larvae under the skin Red, itchy tracts, usually on legs	Penetration of the skin by filariform larvae Penetration of the skin by filariform larvae
Angiostrongylus cantonensis (rat lungworm)	China, Hawaii, and tropical islands	Rat	Eosinophilic meningo-encephalitis	Eosinophilia and symptoms of meningitis, spinal fluid contains many white blood cells including increased eosinophils	Ingestion of infected snail or prawn (intermediate host)
Angiostrongylus costaricensis	Central America	Rat		Adult worms lay eggs in mesenteric arteries near cecum: cause granulomas and abdominal inflammation	Eating unwashed vegetables contaminated with mucous secretions from infected slug (intermediate host)
Anisakis spp. (roundworm of marine mammals and fish)	Japan, Netherlands	Herring, other fish	Eosinophilic granuloma in stomach or small intestine	Abdominal pain and an eosinophilic granuloma around the migrating larvae of *Anisakis* in the intestinal wall	Ingesting raw fish containing the larval stage
Capillariaphilippinensis	Far East	Fish		Malabsorption syndrome; extreme and persistent diarrhea; death due to cardiac failure or secondary infection. Adults multiply in human intestine and cause blockage	Ingestion of infected raw fish

TABLE 2–5. *Continued*

Scientific and Common Name	Geographic Location	Normal Animal Host	Disease	Symptoms in Humans	Method of Infection of Humans
Dirofilaria spp. (filariae of canines)	Various species worldwide	Dog, racoon, fox	***Tropical eosinophilia,*** eosinophilic lung	High eosinophilia, chronic cough, pulmonary infiltrates, high levels of IgE Microfilariae are rarely present in peripheral blood	Bite of mosquito vector carrying infective filaria larvae
Gnathostoma spp.	Far East	Dog, feline		Acute visceral larval migrans syndrome; then intermittent chronic subcutaneous swellings	Ingestion of larva from raw infected fish, or application of infected snake poltice to open lesion; larvae migrate into lesion
Gongylonema pulchrum	Worldwide	Pig		Migrating worm in facial subcutaneous tissue	Accidental ingestion of infected roach or dung beetle
Thelazia spp.	Worldwide	Various mammals		Habitation of conjunctival sac or lacrimal duct by adult. Severe irritation of eye	Contact with infected fly or roach
Toxocara canis; T. cati (large intestinal roundworms of dogs or cats)	Worldwide	Dog, cat	Visceral larval migrans (VLM)	Eosinophilia, hepatomegaly, pulmonary inflammation with cough and fever; possible encystment of the larvae in the eye which mimics a malignant tumor All symptoms due to migration of larvae in the tissues of humans	Ingestion of infective stage larvae in developed eggs from soil

produced in humans following an accidental infection. These parasites do not normally develop full life cycles in humans (although there are exceptions, such as Toxoplasmosis).

You have now completed the chapter covering the Nematoda. After reviewing this material and the related color plates with descriptions, using the learning objectives to direct your studies, proceed to the first post-test. Allow 45 minutes to complete the test. Write your answers on a separate piece of paper. The answers are given in the back of the book. If you score less than 80 percent correct, review all the appropriate material and retake the test. Follow this procedure for all chapter post-tests.

BIBLIOGRAPHY

INTESTINAL NEMATODES

BARRETT-CONNOR, E: *Human intestinal nematodiasis in the United States.* Cal Med 117:8, 1972.

CRUZ, T, REBOUCAS, G, AND ROCHA, H: *Fatal strongyloidiasis in patients receiving corticosteroids.* N Engl J Med 275:1093, 1966.

GLOOR, RF, BREYLERY, ER, AND MARTINEZ, IG: *Hookworm infection in a rural Kentucky county.* Am J Trop Med Hyg 19:1007, 1970.

GOULD, SE: *Trichinosis in Man and Animals.* Charles C Thomas, Springfield, IL, 1970.

GROVE, SS AND ELSDON-DEW, R: *Internal auto-infection with Strongyloides stercoralis.* South Afr J Lab Clin Med 4:55, 1958.

LAYRISSE, M, APARCEDO, L, MARTINEZ-TORRES, C, AND ROCHE, M: *Blood loss due to infection with Trichuris trichiura.* Am J Trop Med Hyg 16:613, 1967.

MARTIN, LK: *Hookworm in Georgia, I. Survey of intestinal helminth infections and anemia in rural school children.* Am J Trop Med Hyg 21:919, 1972.

O'BRIEN, W: *Intestinal malabsorption in acute infection with Strongyloides stercoralis.* Trans Roy Soc Trop Med Hyg 69:69, 1975.

ROCHE, M AND LAYRISSE, M: *The nature and causes of "hookworm anemia."* Am J Trop Med Hyg 15:1031, 1966.

SODEMAN, TM AND DOCK, N: *Laboratory diagnosis of parasitic and fungal diseases of the central nervous system.* Ann Clin Lab Sci 6:47, 1976.

THUNE, O: *Creeping eruption of larval migrans.* Int J Dermatol 11:231, 1972.

FILARIAE

BEVERLEY-BURTON, M AND CRICHTON, VF: *Identification of guinea-worm species.* Trans Roy Soc Trop Med Hyg 67:152, 1973.

CHOYCE, DP: *Epidemiology and natural history of onchocerciasis.* Israel J Med Sci 8:1143, 1972.

CHOYCE, DP: *Onchocerciases: Ophthalmic aspects.* Trans Roy Soc Trop Med Hyg 60:720, 1966.

COOLIDGE, C, ET AL: *Zoonotic Brugia filariasis in New England.* Ann Intern Med 90:341, 1979.

DANARAJ, TJ, PACHECO, G, SHANMUGARATNAM, K, ET AL: *The etiology and pathology of eosinophilic lung (tropical eosinophilia).* Am J Trop Med Hyg 15:183, 1966.

NELSON, GS: *Onchocerciasis.* In DAWES, B (ED): *Advances in Parasitology.* Vol 8. Academic Press, New York, 1970, pp 173–224.

NELSON, GS: *Current concepts in parasitology: Filariasis.* N Engl J Med 300:1136, 1979.

OTTESEN, EA: *Immunopathology of lymphatic filariasis in man.* Springer Seminars in Immunopathology 2:373, 1980.

PRICE, EW: *The mechanism of lymphatic obstruction in endemic elephantiasis of the lower legs.* Trans Roy Soc Trop Med Hyg 69:177, 1975.

Sasa, M: *Human Filariasis.* University Park Press, Baltimore, 1976.

Woodruff, AW: *Toxocariasis.* Br Med J 3:663, 1970.

Zoonoses

Alicata, JE and Jindrak, K: *Angiostrongylosis in the Pacific and Southeast Asia.* Charles C Thomas, Springfield, IL, 1970.

Beaver, PC and Orihel, TC: *Human infection with the filariae of animals in the United States.* Am J Trop Med Hyg 14:1010, 1965.

CRC Handbook Series in Zoonoses, Section C: *Parasitic Zoonoses,* Vols I, II, III. Boca Raton, FL, 1982.

Danz, V, Cabrera, BD, and Canias, B, jr: *Human intestinal capilariasis, 1. Clinical features.* Acta Med Philip 4:72, 1967.

Glickman, LP, et al: *Evaluation of serodiagnostic tests for visceral larval migrans.* Am J Trop Med Hyg 27:492, 1978.

Little, MD and Most, H: *Anisakid larva from the throat of a woman in New York.* Am J Trop Med Hyg 22:609, 1973.

Loría-Cortez, R and Lobo-Sanahija, JF: *Clinical abdominal angiostrongylosis—A study of 116 children with intestinal eosinophilic granuloma caused by A. costaricensis.* Am J Trop Med Hyg 29:538, 1980.

Markell, EK: *Pseudohookworm infection—Trichostrongyliasis. Treatment with thiabendazole.* N Engl J Med 278, 1968.

Meyers, BJ: *The nematodes that cause anasakiasis.* J Milk Food Technol 38:774, 1975.

Morera, P and Cespedes, R: *Angiostrongylus costaricensis n. sp. (Nematoda: Metastrongyloidea): A new lungworm occurring in man in Costa Rica.* Rev Biol Trop 18:173, 1971.

Polnar, GO, Jr and Jansson, HB: *Diseases of Nematodes* (2 vols). CRC Press, Boca Raton, FL, 1988.

Schlotthauer, JC, Harrison, EG, Jr, and Thompson, JH: *Dirofilariasis—An emerging zoonosis?* Arch Environ Health 19:887, 1969.

World Health Organization: *Parasitic Zoonoses.* WHO Technical Report No. 637, Geneva, WHO, 1979.

POST-TEST

1. Draw the life cycle of *Ascaris lumbricoides* in diagram form. Indicate the diagnostic and infective stages. (**10 points**)
2. The following was identified by the night technician. (**15 points**)

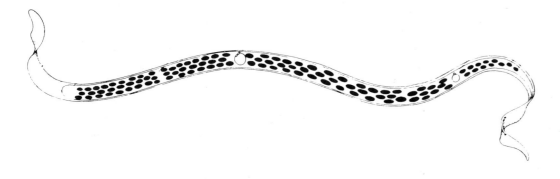

   a. What is the scientific name of the parasite?
   b. What is the intermediate host?
   c. In what body specimen was this organism identified, and what laboratory technique was helpful in finding the organism?

3. Briefly define each of the following: (**25 points**)
   a. cutaneous larval migrans   d. infective stage
   b. diurnal   e. prepatent stage
   c. diagnostic stage

4. For each of the following, fill in the blanks. (**45 points**)

	Common Name	Method of Infection	Body Specimen
Trichuris Trichiura			
Onchocerca volvulus			
Strongyloides stercoralis			
Ancylostoma duodenale			
Enterobius vermicularis			

5. Give the scientific name of three intestinal parasites that can cause a pneumonialike syndrome during the second week after infection. (**5 points**)

3

CESTODA

LEARNING OBJECTIVES

Upon completion of this chapter and its supplementary color plates as described, the student will be able to

1. state the general characteristics of phylum Platyhelminthes.
2. compare and contrast the phylum Nemathelminthes with Platyhelminthes using morphologic criteria.
3. define terminology specifically related to the **Cestoda.**
4. state the scientific and common names of cestodes that parasitize humans.
5. state the methods of diagnosis used to identify cestode infections.
6. describe the general morphology of an adult cestode.
7. describe graphically the general life cycle of a cestode.
8. differentiate adult Cestoda using morphologic criteria.
9. differentiate larval stages of Cestoda using morphologic criteria and/or the required intermediate host.
10. differentiate the diagnostic stages of the Cestoda.
11. discuss the epidemiology and medical importance of cestode zoonoses.
12. given illustrations or photographs (or actual specimens if you have had laboratory experience), identify diagnostic stages of Cestoda and the body specimen of choice to be used for examination for each.
13. identify the stage in the life cycle of each cestode (including the zoonoses) that can parasitize humans.

The Platyhelminthes, as a phylum, are known as the flatworms; these are dorsoventrally flattened and have solid bodies with no body cavity. The internal organs are embedded in tissue called the parenchyma. There are no respiratory or blood-vascular systems. The life cycles of these organisms are generally indirect; that is, at least one intermediate host is required to support larval development.

The two classes of the phylum Platyhelminthes that contain human parasites are the Cestoda (the tapeworms) and the Digenea (the flukes). The Digenea will be covered in chapter 4. Platyhelminthes are all **hermaphroditic** with an important exception: the blood flukes.

The external surface (termed the **tegument**) is highly absorptive and even releases digestive enzymes at its surface from microtriches (specialized microvilli). The digeneans have a rudimentary alimentary tract; some nutrients are taken in by mouth and some are absorbed through the tegument. The cestodes, on the other hand, must absorb all nutrients through the tegument because this class of parasites has no mouth or digestive tract.

TABLE 3–1. Cestoda

Order	Scientific Name	Common Name
Cyclophyllidae	*Hymenolepis nana* (high"men-ol'e-pis/nay'nuh)	dwarf tapeworm
Cyclophyllidae	*Taenia saginata* (tee'nee-uh/sadj-i-nay'tuh)	beef tapeworm
Cyclophillidae	*Taenia solium* (tee'nee-uh/so-lee'um)	pork tapeworm
Cyclophillidae	*Echinococcus granulosus* (eh-kigh"no-kock'us/gran-yoo-lo'sus)	dog tapeworm, hydatid tapeworm
Pseudophyllidae	*Diphyllobothrium latum* (dye-fil"o-both-ree-um/lay'tum)	broad fish tapeworm

Members of the class **Cestoda** are commonly called tapeworms, inasmuch as they are long and ribbonlike and are flattened in cross-section. The body of the tapeworm consists of segments known as **proglottids.** The adult may range from a few millimeters to 20 meters in length, depending on the species. The adult cestode lives in the intestinal tract of the vertebrate definitive host, while the larval stage inhabits tissues of the intermediate host.

The anterior end of the worm (termed **scolex**) is modified for attachment to the intestinal wall of the definitive host. The scolex is usually equipped with four cup-shaped suckers, and some species also have a crown of hooks on the scolex to aid in attachment. A scolex is less than 2 mm long even though the whole tapeworm can be 20 m in body length. These worms have no mouth, digestive tract, or vascular system, and all nutrients are absorbed through the outer surface of the body. Waste products are released through the tegument as well. The entire body of an adult tapeworm is termed the strobila. Segments form by budding from the posterior end of the scolex, an area of germinal tissue for new segment production.

Each tapeworm is hermaphroditic. Every mature proglottid of the body contains both male and female reproductive organs. The sex organs in each proglottid mature gradually so that the proglottids at the terminus of the tapeworm contain fully developed reproductive organs and the uterus is filled with fertilized eggs. These posterior segments are termed gravid proglottids. The embryo seen in tapeworm eggs (termed the **onchosphere** or **hexacanth embryo**) bears six tiny hooklets, which facilitate entry of the embryo into the intestinal mucosa of the intermediate host.

In Table 3–1 are listed the scientific names (genus and species) and the common names for the cestodes of medical importance. Use the pronunciation guide and repeat each name to yourself several times. On the following pages are shown the life-cycle diagrams of these tapeworms, and Table 3–2 reviews the pertinent information on tapeworms. Proceed to the post-test when you have learned the vocabulary and the introductory material and have mastered the life cycles, color plates, and review table.

GLOSSARY

Cestoda. A class within the phylum *Platyhelminthes,* which includes the tapeworms. These helminths have elongated, ribbonlike, segmented bodies.

anaphylaxis (anaphylactic shock). An exaggerated histamine-release reaction by the host's body to foreign protein, allergen, or other substances; may be fatal.

anorexia. Loss of appetite.

brood capsule. A structure within the daughter cyst in *Echinococcus granulosus* in which many scolices grow. Each scolex could develop into an adult tapeworm in the definitive host.

coracidium. A ciliated hexacanth embryo; *Diphyllobothrium latum* eggs develop to this stage and hatch in fresh water.

cysticercoid. The larval stage of some tapeworms (e.g., *Hymenolepis nana*); a small, bladderlike structure containing little or no fluid in which the scolex is enclosed.

cysticercus. A thin-walled, fluid-filled, bladderlike cyst that encloses a scolex. Also termed a bladder worm, larvae develop in this form (e.g., *Taenia* spp.).

embryophore. The shell of *Taenia* and other tapeworm eggs as these are seen in feces.

hermaphroditic. Having both male and female reproductive organs within the same individual. All tapeworms have both sets of reproductive organs in each segment of the adult.

hexacanth embryo. A tapeworm larva having six hooklets (see **onchosphere**).

hydatid cyst. A vesicular structure formed by *E. granulosus* larvae in the intermediate host; contains fluid, brood capsules, and also daughter cysts in which the scolices of potential tapeworms are formed.

hydatid sand. Granular material consisting of free scolices, hooklets, daughter cysts, and amorphous material. Found in the fluid of older cysts of *E. granulosus*.

onchosphere. The motile, first-stage larva of certain cestodes armed with six hooklets (also termed hexacanth embryo).

operculum. The lid or caplike cover on certain platyhelminth eggs (e.g., *Diphyllobothrium latum*).

plerocercoid. The larval stage in the development of *D. latum* that develops after the procercoid stage is ingested by a freshwater fish. This form has an immature scolex and is infective if eaten by humans.

procercoid. The larval stage that develops from the coracidium of *D. latum*. It develops in the body of a freshwater crustacean.

proglottid. One of the segments of a tapeworm. Each proglottid contains male and female reproductive organs when mature.

racemose. Clusters with branching, nodular terminations resembling a bunch of grapes. Used in reference to larval cysticercosis caused by the migration and development of *T. solium* larvae in the brain tissue of humans. An aberrant form.

rostellum. The fleshy anterior protuberance of the scolex of some tapeworms (species specific); may bear a circular row (or rows) of hooks; may be retractable.

scolex (pl. **scolices**). Anterior end of a tapeworm; causes attachment to the wall of the intestine of a host by means of suckers and sometimes hooks.

sparganosis. Pleurocercoid in human tissue from accidental infection with procercoid.

tegument (integument). The absorptive body surface of platyhelminths.

transport host. Vector; often a blood-sucking insect.

viscera (sing. **viscus**). Any of the large organs in the interior of any of the four great body cavities of vertebrates.

DIAGRAM 3–1. *Hymenolepis nana* (dwarf tapeworm)

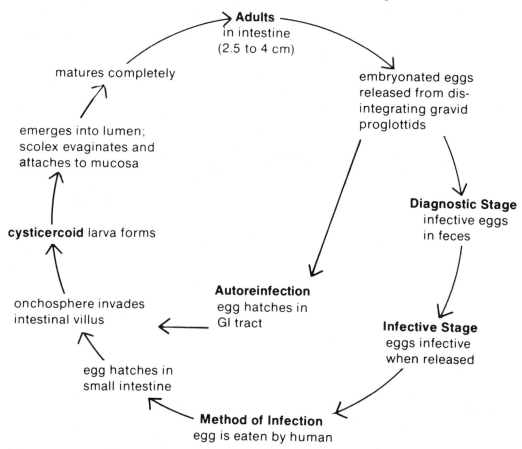

Adults
in intestine
(2.5 to 4 cm)

matures completely

embryonated eggs
released from dis-
integrating gravid
proglottids

emerges into lumen;
scolex evaginates and
attaches to mucosa

Diagnostic Stage
infective eggs
in feces

cysticercoid larva forms

onchosphere invades
intestinal villus

Autoreinfection
egg hatches in
GI tract

Infective Stage
eggs infective
when released

egg hatches in
small intestine

Method of Infection
egg is eaten by human

METHOD OF DIAGNOSIS

Recovery and identification of eggs in feces.

DIAGNOSTIC STAGE

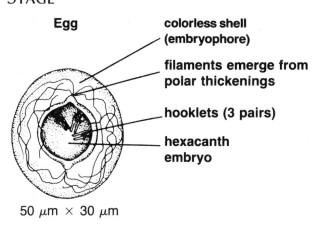

Egg

colorless shell
(embryophore)

filaments emerge from
polar thickenings

hooklets (3 pairs)

hexacanth
embryo

50 μm × 30 μm

DISEASE NAME

Dwarf tapeworm infection

MAJOR PATHOLOGY AND SYMPTOMS

1. light infection—asymptomatic
2. heavy infection—intestinal enteritis; abdominal pain, diarrhea, headache, dizziness, anorexia
3. multiple infections are common

TREATMENT

1. praziquantel
2. niclosamide

DISTRIBUTION

Worldwide, tropics and subtropics, especially in children and in institutionalized persons living in close quarters. Most common human tapeworm in the U.S., with greater prevalence in the Southeast, where 3 percent infection is estimated.

OF NOTE

1. The dwarf tapeworm requires no intermediate host, but fleas and beetles can serve as **transport hosts. Cysticercoid** larvae can develop in the body cavity of these insects and are infective to either humans or rodents if accidentally ingested.
2. Eggs in feces from infected mice and rats are a common source of human infection.

DIAGRAM 3–2. *Taenia saginata* (beef tapeworm) and *Taenia solium* (pork tapeworm)

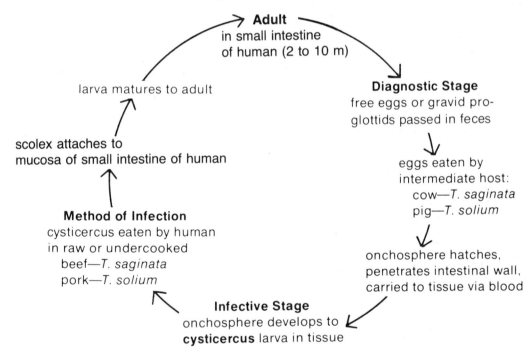

METHOD OF DIAGNOSIS

Recovery of egg or gravid proglottid (or scolex after drug treatment) in feces. For specific proglottid and scolex identification: *T. saginata* has 15 to 30 lateral uterine branches in the gravid proglottid and a scolex with only four suckers; *T. solium* has a gravid proglottid with 7 to 12 lateral uterine branches, and the scolex has four suckers with a central crown of hooks. *T. solium* is called the "armed" tapeworm because of the crown of hooks by which the scolex attaches to the intestinal wall. (See Color Plate 40.) The eggs of these two species are identical.

Immunologic Methods

For cysticercosis: ELISA; indirect hemagglutination

Diagnostic Stage

Intact gravid proglottids may be found and must be differentiated. (See Color Plates 42 and 43.)

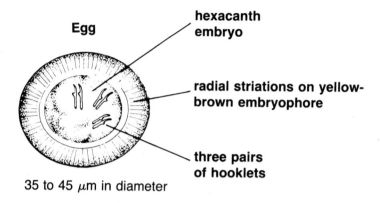

35 to 45 μm in diameter

Disease Names

T. saginata: taeniasis, beef tapeworm infection
T. solium: taeniasis, pork tapeworm infection

Major Pathology and Symptoms

1. Most infected people are asymptomatic. Abdominal pain, diarrhea, and weight loss can occur.
2. Man can serve as an intermediate host for *Taenia solium*. If eggs of *T. solium* are accidentally ingested, or if eggs are released from a proglottid in the intestinal tract, the eggs can hatch in the intestine, and the larvae will migrate to form cysticercus cysts in any organ or nervous tissue (cysticercosis). This can be fatal if the **racemose** form develops in the brain.

Treatment

For adult: niclosamide.
For cysticercosis: praziquantel; surgery.

Distribution

T. saginata—cosmopolitan in countries where beef is eaten raw or insufficiently cooked. Found in Southwest U.S.
T. solium—cosmopolitan where pork is eaten raw or undercooked.

Of Note

1. Humans are the only known definitive host for these *Taenias*.
2. The adult worms live for many years and usually only one worm is present.
3. Human cysticercosis is common in Mexico and Central America.

DIAGRAM 3–3. *Diphyllobothrium latum* (broad fish tapeworm)

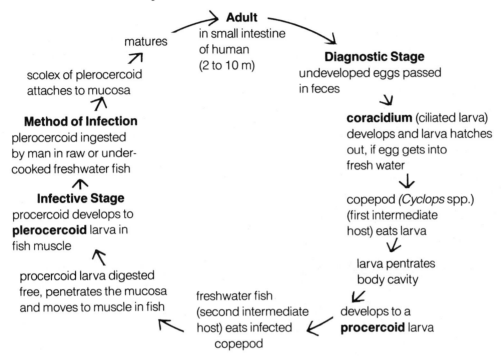

matures → **Adult** in small intestine of human (2 to 10 m)

scolex of plerocercoid attaches to mucosa

Method of Infection plerocercoid ingested by man in raw or under-cooked freshwater fish

Infective Stage procercoid develops to **plerocercoid** larva in fish muscle

procercoid larva digested free, penetrates the mucosa and moves to muscle in fish

freshwater fish (second intermediate host) eats infected copepod

Diagnostic Stage undeveloped eggs passed in feces

coracidium (ciliated larva) develops and larva hatches out, if egg gets into fresh water

copepod *(Cyclops* spp.) (first intermediate host) eats larva

larva pentrates body cavity

develops to a **procercoid** larva

METHOD OF DIAGNOSIS

Recovery of eggs in feces. Evacuated proglottids and scolices are also diagnostic in feces but are rarely naturally evacuated intact.

DIAGNOSTIC STAGE

Egg

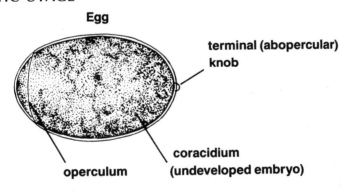

terminal (abopercular) knob

operculum

coracidium (undeveloped embryo)

75 μm × 45 μm

DISEASE NAMES

Diphyllobothriasis, dibothriocephalus anemia, fish tapeworm infection, broadfish tapeworm infection.

MAJOR PATHOLOGY AND SYMPTOMS

1. Intestinal obstruction (adult can grow to 20 m) and abdominal pain. Most infected persons exhibit vague digestive symptoms.
2. Weight loss and weakness.
3. Anemia (macrocytic type) and eventual nervous system disturbances due to a B_{12} deficiency caused by the tapeworm's utilization of up to 100 percent dietary B_{12} in about 1 percent of infected persons; usually restricted to persons of Scandinavian descent.

TREATMENT

Niclosamide or praziquantel

DISTRIBUTION

Temperate regions where freshwater fish are a common part of the diet, or where raw fish are eaten (the U.S. Great Lakes region, Alaska, Chile, Argentina, Central Africa, and parts of Asia). In Europe, estimates of infection include 20 percent of the Finnish people and up to 100 percent in the Baltic region.

OF NOTE

1. Usually only one adult is present.
2. A variety of fish-eating mammals can serve as definitive hosts, in addition to humans.
3. The procercoid may be passed up the food chain in a dormant condition through small to larger game fish (e.g., Northern or walleyed pike).
4. A human can harbor a tissue plerocercoid if a procercoid in a copepod is ingested (see Sparganosis, page 45).
5. Feces must be screened after drug treatment to assure passage of the scolex so that no new proglottids will be formed. **N.B.** If niclosamide is used the scolex will not be recovered.

DIAGRAM 3–4. *Echinococcus granulosus* (hydatid tapeworm)

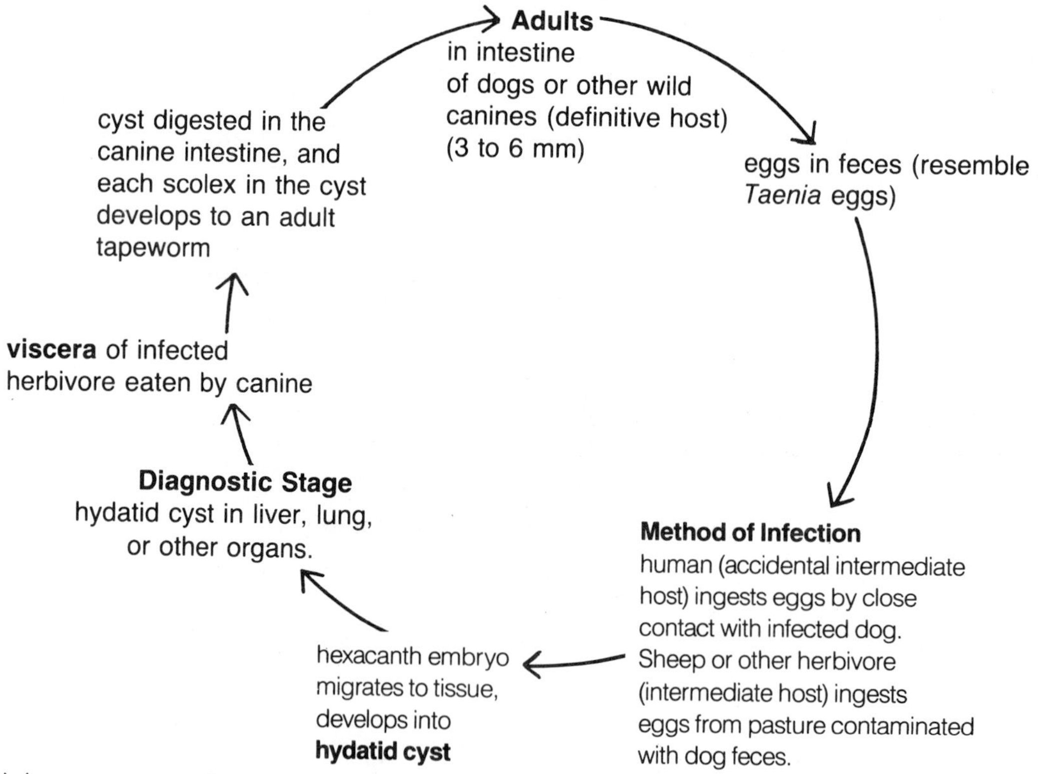

Adults
in intestine
of dogs or other wild
canines (definitive host)
(3 to 6 mm)

eggs in feces (resemble *Taenia* eggs)

cyst digested in the canine intestine, and each scolex in the cyst develops to an adult tapeworm

viscera of infected herbivore eaten by canine

Diagnostic Stage
hydatid cyst in liver, lung, or other organs.

hexacanth embryo migrates to tissue, develops into **hydatid cyst**

Method of Infection
human (accidental intermediate host) ingests eggs by close contact with infected dog. Sheep or other herbivore (intermediate host) ingests eggs from pasture contaminated with dog feces.

METHOD OF DIAGNOSIS

1. Serologic tests.
2. Presence of scolices, **brood capsules, hydatid sand,** or daughter cysts in the hydatid cyst fluid as detected by biopsy (not recommended because leakage of cyst fluid can cause **anaphylaxis**).
3. X-ray or ultrasound scan detection of cyst mass in organ, especially if calcified.

DIAGNOSTIC STAGE

Hydatid cyst (partial cross-section)

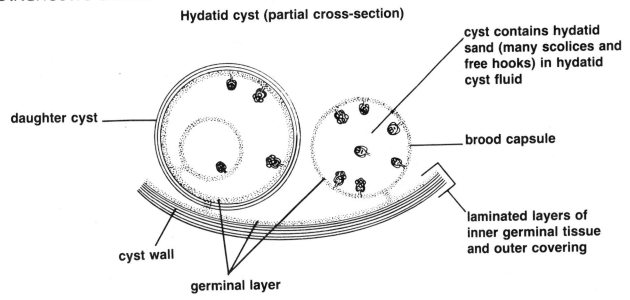

daughter cyst

cyst contains hydatid sand (many scolices and free hooks) in hydatid cyst fluid

brood capsule

laminated layers of inner germinal tissue and outer covering

cyst wall

germinal layer

DISEASE NAMES

Echinococcosis, hydatid cyst, hydatid disease, hydatidosis

MAJOR PATHOLOGY AND SYMPTOMS

1. Vary according to location and size of cyst.
    a. in liver (most common site)—no symptoms until cyst gets large (close to a year after ingestion of egg); can cause jaundice or portal hypertension.
    b. in lung—no symptoms until cyst gets large; coughing, shortness of breath, chest pain.
    c. other sites—symptoms related to enlarging cyst.
2. Cyst growth or rupture can result in death.
3. Anaphylactic shock if cyst ruptures (may occur during biopsy procedure).
4. Eosinophilia, urticaria, bronchospasm.

TREATMENT

1. Surgery
2. Mebendazole or albendazole

DISTRIBUTION

Cosmopolitan; human infections primarily in sheep-raising areas where domestic dogs are used in herding.

OF NOTE

1. Hydatid disease in the U.S. is reported mainly in the Southwest, chiefly among the Navaho Indians and in Utah, Alaska, and Canada.
2. *E. multilocularis,* which forms alveolar cysts, is more rare in humans but is intensely pathogenic and generally fatal without treatment.

TABLE 3–2. (A) Human Infections with Cestoda

Scientific and Common Name	Epidemiology	Disease Producing Form and Its Location in Host	How Human Infection Occurs	Major Disease Manifestations, Diagnostic Stage, and Specimen of Choice
Hymenolepis nana (dwarf tapeworm)	Worldwide (common in southeastern U.S.)	Adults live in small intestine	Egg ingested by man in contaminated food or water or hand to mouth; autoinfection is common.	Light infections—asymptomatic; heavy worm burdens cause abdominal pain, diarrhea, headaches, dizziness. Diagnosis: eggs in feces
Taenia saginata (beef tapeworm)	Cosmopolitan in beef-eating countries	Adult lives in small intestine	*Cysticercus bovis* larva eaten by human in undercooked beef	Most people are asymptomatic. Can experience abdominal pain, diarrhea, weight loss. Diagnosis: eggs or proglottid in feces
Taenia solium	Worldwide (rare in U.S.)	Adult lives in small intestine	*Cysticercus cellulosa* larva eaten by human in undercooked pork	Same as *Taenia saginata*
Diphyllobothrium latum	Temperate areas where freshwater fish is eaten undercooked or raw	Adult lives in small intestine	Plerocercoid larva ingested by humans in freshwater fish	Can cause intestinal obstruction and macrocytic anemia due to B_{12} deficiency; abdominal pain and weight loss

(B) Accidental Zoonotic Human Infections with Cestoda

Scientific and Common Name	Epidemiology	Disease Producing Form and Its Location in Host	How Human Infection Occurs	Major Disease Manifestations, Diagnostic Stage, and Specimen of Choice
Echinococcus granulosus (dog tapeworm)	Worldwide in sheep-raising areas	Adult lives in the intestine of dogs or other wild canines	Human accidentally ingests eggs by close contact with infected dog; usual intermediate host—sheep	Cyst can be found in the liver (most commonly) or lung of man. Lung symptoms include coughing and pain. Leakage

TABLE 3–2. (B) *Continued*

Scientific and Common Name	Epidemiology	Disease Producing Form and Its Location in Host	How Human Infection Occurs	Major Disease Manifestations, Diagnostic Stage, and Specimen of Choice
				of hydatid fluid causes allergy and eosinophilia. Diagnosis: X-ray, serology
Hymenolepis diminuta (rat tapeworm)	Worldwide	Adult lives in the intestine; usual host of adult tapeworm is the rat	Human accidentally ingests cysticercoid larva in infected flea or grain beetle (intermediate host)	Mild symptoms; tapeworms are frequently lost spontaneously. Eggs in feces are diagnostic.
Dipylidium caninum (dog or cat)	Worldwide	Adult lives in the intestine; usual host of adult tapeworm is the dog or cat	Human accidentally ingests cysticercoid larva in infected dog or cat flea (intermediate host). Rare, occurs mainly in children	Mild intestinal disturbances. Tapeworms are frequently lost spontaneously. Egg packets or proglottids are diagnostic in feces.
Sparganosis (*Diphyllobothrium* or *Spirometra* spp.)	Far East freshwater areas	Plerocercoid in tissues	Human accidentally ingests copepod containing a procercoid.	Subcutaneous nodules or internal abscesses or cysts
Cysticercosis (*Taenia solium*)	Cosmopolitan	Cysticercoid larva in human tissue; usual host of larva is pig	Human accidentally ingests egg, or eggs, released from proglottid of adult in human intestine	2 cm painless swelling if in skin; pain and other symptoms if in eye; seizures or other neurologic symptoms or death if in brain

You have now completed the section on the *Cestoda*. After reviewing this material with the aid of your learning objectives, proceed to the post-test.

BIBLIOGRAPHY

COLTORTI, EA AND VARELA-DIAZ, VM: *Detection of antibodies against granulosus are five antigens by double diffusion test.* Trans Roy Soc Trop Med Hyg 72:227, 1978.

LEIBY, PD AND KRITSKY, DL: *Echinococcus multilocularis: A possible domestic life cycle in central North America and its public health importance.* J Parasitol 58:1213, 1972.

SCHWABE, CW, RUPPANNER, R, MILLER, CW, ET AL: *Hydatid disease is endemic in California.* Cal Med 117:13, 1972.

SMYTH, JD: *The biology of the hydatid organism.* In DAWES, B (ED): *Advances in Parasitology*, Vol 2. Academic Press, New York, 1964, pp. 169–219.

VON BONDSDORFF, B: *Diphyllobothriasis in man.* Academic Press, New York, 1977.

POST-TEST

1. Define and cite an example of each of the following: (**20 points**)
   a. hexacanth embryo
   b. hermaphroditic
   c. "armed" scolex
   d. proglottid
   e. hydatid cyst

2. Matching: select correct intermediate host(s) for each parasite: (**20 points**)
   a. _5_ *Taenia solium*
   b. _9_ *Hymenolepis nana*
   c. _7_ *Dipylidium caninum*
   d. _2,1_ *Diphyllobothrium latum*
   e. _10,4_ *Echinococcus granulosus*

   1. fish
   2. copepod
   3. cow
   4. human
   5. pig
   6. snail
   7. flea
   8. dog
   9. none
   10. sheep

3. Draw and label the diagnostic stage(s) for each of the following as you would observe them microscopically in human feces: (**50 points**)
   a. dwarf tapeworm
   b. broad fish tapeworm
   c. beef tapeworm
   d. pork tapeworm
   e. hydatid cyst

4. Matching: Select one only: (**10 points**)
   a. _6_ *Taenia solium*
   b. _2_ *Taenia saginata*
   c. _5_ *Hymenolepis nana*
   d. _1_ *Diphyllobothrium latum*
   e. _8_ *Echinococcus granulosus*
   f. _7_ *Dipylidium caninum*
   g. _3_ *Sparganosis*
   h. _4_ *Cysticercosis*

   1. macrocytic anemia, vitamin B_{12} deficiency
   2. scolex lacks crown of hooks
   3. pleurocercoid subcutaneously
   4. neurologic symptoms if in brain
   5. autoreinfection is common
   6. proglottid has 7–10 lateral uterine branches
   7. human accidentally ingests infected flea
   8. cysts found in liver, lungs or other organs

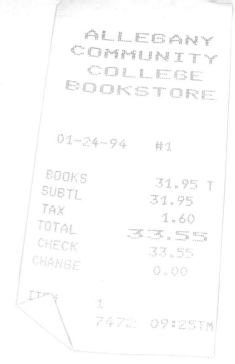

DIGENEA

LEARNING OBJECTIVES

Upon completion of this chapter and its supplementary color plates as described, the student will be able to

1. define terminology specific for flukes.
2. state scientific and common names of flukes that parasitize humans.
3. describe the general morphology of an adult hermaphroditic Digenea.
4. describe the general morphology of adult schistosomes.
5. describe graphically the life cycle of adult trematodes.
6. state the methods of diagnosis used to identify fluke infections.
7. differentiate adult Digenea using morphologic criteria.
8. differentiate diagnostic stages of Digenea.
9. classify the methods by which the flukes infect humans.
10. compare and contrast the morphology of adult Cestoda and Digenea.
11. given an illustration or photograph (or an actual specimen if you have had laboratory experience), identify diagnostic stages of Digenea and the body specimen of choice to be used for examination for each.
12. discriminate between the Digenea on the basis of required intermediate host(s).

Digenea (commonly called flukes) belong to the phylum Platyhelminthes along with the Cestoda. Flukes in the class Digenea (includes parasites in humans) are flattened dorsoventrally and are nonsegmented, leaf-shaped helminths. Parasitic species inhabit the intestine or tissues of humans. Digenea vary in size from a few millimeters to several

TABLE 4–1. Hermaphroditic Flukes

Order	Scientific Name	Common Name
Echinostomida	*Fasciolopsis buski* (fa-see'o-lop'sis/bus'kee)	large intestinal fluke
Echinostomida	*Fasciola hepatica* (fa-see'o-luh/he-pat'i-kuh)	sheep liver fluke
Opisthorchiida	*Clonorchis sinensis* (klo-nor'kis/si-nen'sis)	Chinese liver fluke
Opisthorchiida	*Heterophyes heterophyes* (het-ur-off'ee-eez/het"ur-off'ee-eez)	heterophid fluke
Opisthorchiida	*Metagonimus yokogawai* (met'uh-gon'i-mus/yo-ko-gah-wah'eye)	heterophid fluke
Plagiorchiida	*Paragonimus westermani* (par"i-gon-'i-mus/wes-tur-man'eye)	Oriental lung fluke

TABLE 4–2. Blood Flukes

Order	Scientific Name	Common Name
Strigeatida	*Schistosoma mansoni* (shis'to-so'muh/man-so'nigh)	Manson's blood fluke
Strigeatida	*Schistosoma japonicum* (shis'to-so'muh/ja-pon'i-kum)	blood fluke
Strigeatida	*Schistosoma haematobium* (shis'to-so'muh/hee-muh-toe'bee-um)	bladder fluke

centimeters in length. All adult flukes have two cup-shaped muscular suckers (**acetabula**)—an oral sucker and a ventral sucker. The digestive system is simple; the oral cavity is in the center of the oral sucker, and the intestinal tract ends blindly in one or two sacs. There is no anal opening, and waste products are regurgitated. The body surface (tegument) of the fluke is metabolically active, as is true for the Cestoda, and can absorb soluble nutrients and release soluble waste products at the surface.

There are two types of parasitic flukes that can be present in humans. One type lives in the intestine or in other host organs and is hermaphroditic, having both sets of complex, highly branched reproductive organs in each adult fluke. These flukes are listed in Table 4–1. The second type are flukes that live as unisexual adult male and female organisms in the blood vessels of the definitive host. These are known as the *Schistosoma*. The body of the male schistosome curves up along the lateral edges and forms a long channel (the gynecophoral canal) which wraps around the female worm. They coexist in pairs during their adult lifespan in the blood vessels. These flukes are listed separately in Table 4–2. In both types, sexual reproduction in the adult *Digenea* in humans is followed by asexual multiplication of the larval stages harbored by a specific species of snail (a required intermediate host for all flukes).

The life cycles of the flukes are complex (see Diagram 4–1). The adult fluke lays eggs that leave the definitive host via feces, urine, or sputum (depending upon the species and host location of the adult fluke). A specific freshwater species of snail is required as an intermediate host for each species of fluke. In general, the life cycle is as follows: the larval stage (a ciliated **miracidium**) emerges from the egg in fresh water, enters the snail host, and undergoes several cycles of asexual multiplication. The final larval stage leaving the snail is known as the **cercaria**. Many hundreds of cercariae result from each miracidium that enters the snail host. Motile schistosome (blood fluke) cercariae then directly penetrate the tissues of humans when contacting cercaria in infested fresh water. However, the cercariae of the hermaphroditic flukes secrete a thick wall and encyst as a **metacercaria** on aquatic vegetation, or they can enter a second intermediate host (a freshwater fish or crustacean). Only a few species of fish or crustaceans may serve as the second intermediate host for each species of hermaphroditic fluke. Human infection by these hermaphroditic flukes occurs, therefore, when humans eat uncooked water vegetation or the second intermediate host containing the encysted form of the larva (metacercaria).

DIAGRAM 4–1. General life cycles of Trematoda

(A) General Life Cycles of Organ-Dwelling Flukes

Adult Organ Fluke

A. in intestine
  1. *Fasciolopsis buski*
  2. *Heterophyes heterophyes*
B. in bile duct
  3. *Fasciola hepatica*
  4. *Clonorchis sinensis*
C. in lung
  5. *Paragonimus westermani*
(all are hermaphroditic)

excysted metacercaria migrates to appropriate site and matures to adult stage

metacercaria digested free in intestinal tract and excysts

Method of Infection
human eats plant, fish, or crab containing encysted metacercariae

Infective Stage
cercariae encyst on water plant as metacercariae (**1** and **3**), or cercariae enter second intermediate host and encyst in tissue as metacercariae (**2** and **4**—in fish; **5**—in crab or crayfish)

Diagnostic Stage
eggs leave host in:
  1 to **5**—feces or
  5—sputum

in fresh water, eggs develop; miracidium hatches from egg

miracidium penetrates snail (specific species; first intermediate host)

miracidium develops to a **sporocyst**

many **rediae** produced inside sporocyst

rediae develop and produce many cercariae

cercariae emerge from snail

DIAGRAM 4–1. (cont.)

(B) General Life Cycle of Blood Flukes

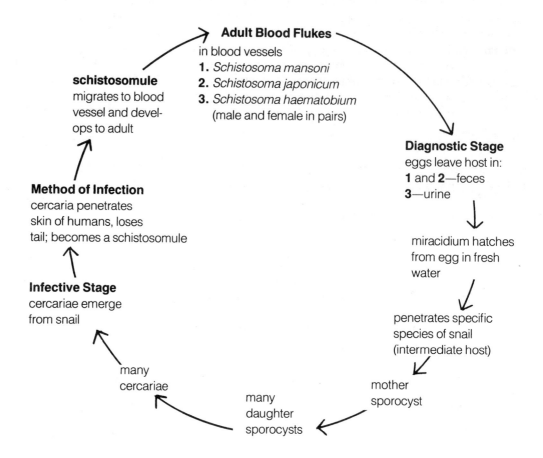

GLOSSARY

DIGENEA. A class of the phylum Platyhelminthes which includes the flukes (trematodes). These have flattened, leaf-shaped bodies bearing muscular suckers. Many species are hermaphroditic.

acetabula (sing. **acetabulum**). Muscular suckers found on the ventral surface of the flukes.

cercaria (pl. **cercariae**). The stage of the fluke life cycle that develops from germ cells in a daughter sporocyst or redia. This is the final development stage in the snail host, consisting of a body and a tail that aids in swimming after it leaves the snail.

distomiasis. Infection with flukes.

granuloma. A tumor or growth of lymphoid or other cells around a foreign body.

metacercaria (pl. **metacercariae**). The stage of the hermaphroditic fluke life cycle occurring when a cercaria has shed its tail, secreted a protective wall, and encysted as a resting stage on water plants or in a second intermediate host; infective stage for humans.

miracidium (pl. **miracidia**). Ciliated first-stage, free-swimming larva of a Digenea, which emerges from the egg and must penetrate the appropriate species of snail in order to continue its life cycle.

redia. The second or third larval stage of a trematode which develops within a sporocyst. Elongated, saclike organisms with a mouth and a gut. Many rediae develop in one sporocyst. Each redia gives rise to many of the next trematode larval stage, the cercariae.

Schistosoma. A genus of *Digenea*, commonly called the blood flukes. They have an elongated shape, separate sexes, and are found in the blood vessels of their definitive host.

schistosomule. The immature schistosome in human tissues after the cercaria has lost the tail during penetration of skin.

sporocyst. The larval form of a trematode which develops from a miracidium in the snail intermediate host. It forms a simple saclike structure containing germinal cells that bud off internally and continue a process of larval multiplication, producing many rediae in each sporocyst.

DIAGRAM 4–2. *Fasciolopsis buski* (large intestinal fluke) and *Fasciola hepatica* (sheep liver fluke)

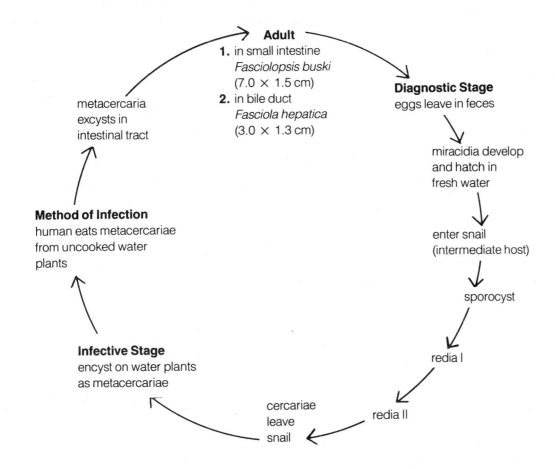

METHOD OF DIAGNOSIS

Recovery of eggs in feces. Eggs of these two species are too similar to differentiate. Species diagnosis depends on clinical signs, travel history, and/or recovery of adult *Fasciolopsis*.

DIAGNOSTIC STAGE

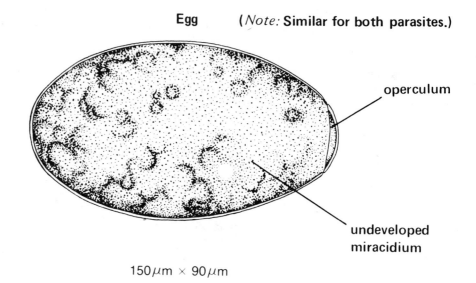

Egg (*Note:* Similar for both parasites.)

operculum

undeveloped
miracidium

150μm × 90μm

DISEASE NAMES

F. buski = fasciolopsiasis; *F. hepatica* = sheep liver rot

MAJOR PATHOLOGY AND SYMPTOMS

1. *F. buski*—mucosal ulcers and hypersecretion around worm attachment site, pain, nausea, mucous diarrhea, anemia, intestinal obstruction and malabsorption, generalized edema, and marked eosinophilia in heavy infections; can cause death.
2. *F. hepatica*—fever, hepatomegaly, and eosinophilia in endemic areas suggest clinical diagnosis. Jaundice, bile duct obstruction, diarrhea, and anemia may occur in severe infection. Pruritis, urticaria, cough.

TREATMENT

F. buski: (1) praziquantel or niclosamide, (2) tetra-chloroethylene
F. hepatica: bithionol

DISTRIBUTION

F. buski—Eastern Asia and Southwest Pacific;
F. hepatica—Cosmopolitan distribution in sheep- and cattle-raising countries; uncommon in the United States.

OF NOTE

1. The natural definitive host for *Fasciola hepatica* is the sheep; therefore, infection of humans is a zoonotic disease. *Fasciolopsis buski* is common in pigs.

DIAGRAM 4–3. *Clonorchis sinensis* (Oriental or Chinese liver fluke; *Opisthorchis*)

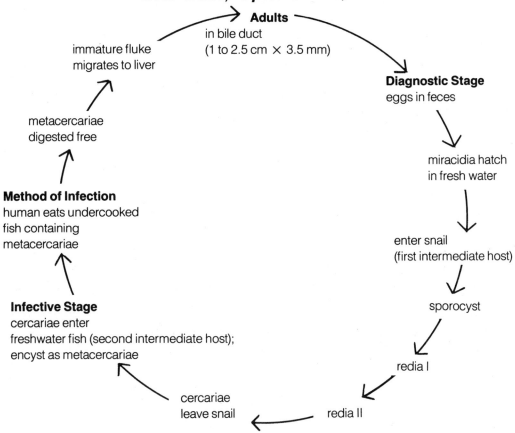

Adults
in bile duct
(1 to 2.5 cm × 3.5 mm)

immature fluke
migrates to liver

metacercariae
digested free

Method of Infection
human eats undercooked
fish containing
metacercariae

Infective Stage
cercariae enter
freshwater fish (second intermediate host);
encyst as metacercariae

cercariae
leave snail

redia II

redia I

sporocyst

enter snail
(first intermediate host)

miracidia hatch
in fresh water

Diagnostic Stage
eggs in feces

METHOD OF DIAGNOSIS

Recovery and identification of eggs in feces or biliary drainage. Radiographic studies.

DIAGNOSTIC STAGE

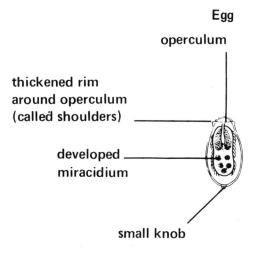

Egg

operculum

thickened rim
around operculum
(called shoulders)

developed
miracidium

small knob

30 μm × 16 μm

DISEASE NAME

Clonorchiasis

Major Pathology and Symptoms

1. light infections may be symptomless
2. jaundice due to bile duct pathology
3. hepatomegaly with tenderness in upper right quadrant
4. abdominal pain and diarrhea, anorexia
5. chronic cases with heavy worm burden from repeated infections may induce severe hepatic complications; rarely, pancreatitis, bile duct stones, cholangitis, cholangiocarcinoma

Treatment

Praziquantel

Distribution

Far East, especially South China

Of Note

Eggs are passed intermittently; therefore, do repeated stool examinations.

DIAGRAM 4–4. *Heterophyes heterophyes* and *Metagonimus yokogawai* (heterophyid)

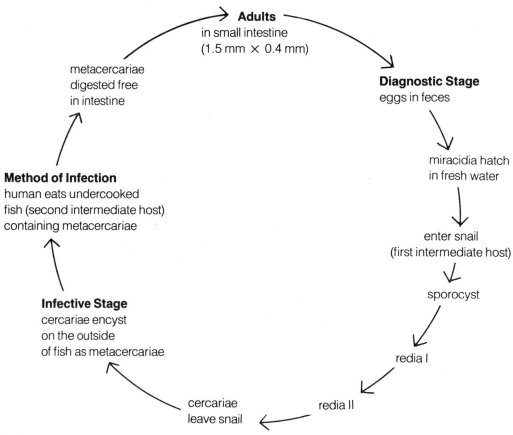

Method of Diagnosis

Recovery and identification of eggs in feces. Difficult to differentiate. (Lack knob at end opposite operculum, which is seen on *C. sinensis* eggs)

DIAGNOSTIC STAGE

(*Note:* **Similar for both parasites but easily confused with** *Clonorchis sinensis*.)

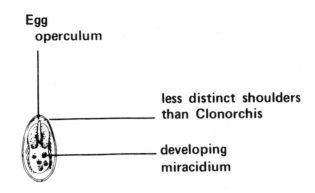

Egg
operculum

less distinct shoulders than Clonorchis

developing miracidium

30μm × 16μm

DISEASE NAMES

H. heterophyes—Heterophyiasis; *M. yokogawai*—Metagonimiasis

MAJOR PATHOLOGY AND SYMPTOMS

Asymptomatic unless harboring a heavy infection which may induce a chronic mucous diarrhea and abdominal pain

TREATMENT

Praziquantel

DISTRIBUTION

H. heterophyes—Near East, Far East, parts of Africa; *M. yokogawai*—Asia and Siberia

OF NOTE

1. Primarily parasites of dogs, cats, and other carnivores.
2. Eggs may travel into tissues, causing granulomas and tissue disorders.
3. *H. heterophyes* has a third sucker around the genital opening.

DIAGRAM 4–5. *Paragonimus westermani* (Oriental lung fluke)

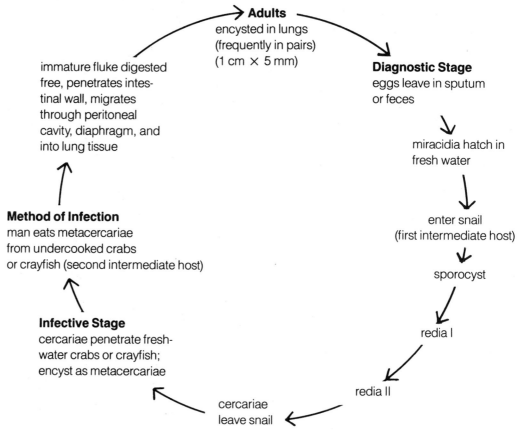

Adults
encysted in lungs
(frequently in pairs)
(1 cm × 5 mm)

immature fluke digested
free, penetrates intes-
tinal wall, migrates
through peritoneal
cavity, diaphragm, and
into lung tissue

Diagnostic Stage
eggs leave in sputum
or feces

miracidia hatch in
fresh water

enter snail
(first intermediate host)

sporocyst

redia I

redia II

cercariae
leave snail

Method of Infection
man eats metacercariae
from undercooked crabs
or crayfish (second intermediate host)

Infective Stage
cercariae penetrate freshwater crabs or crayfish;
encyst as metacercariae

METHOD OF DIAGNOSIS

Recovery and identification of eggs in bloody sputum (resemble iron filings) or in feces; x-ray of lungs; serology: ELISA.

DIAGNOSTIC STAGE

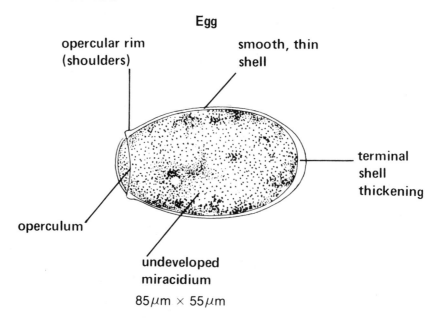

Egg

opercular rim
(shoulders)

smooth, thin
shell

operculum

terminal
shell
thickening

undeveloped
miracidium

85 μm × 55 μm

DISEASE NAMES

Paragonimiasis, pulmonary distomiasis

MAJOR PATHOLOGY AND SYMPTOMS

1. Chronic chest pain, cough, blood-tinged sputum (rusty sputum); lung infiltration, nodules, abscesses; adults present in fibrous cysts, eggs pass through cysts and rupture into bronchioles. Chest x-ray may resemble tuberculosis.
2. Cerebral paragonimiasis causes symptoms of a space-occupying lesion. Abdominal paragonimiasis is usually asymptomatic but common.

TREATMENT

1. Praziquantel
2. Bithional

DISTRIBUTION

Most common in the Far East; also found in parts of Africa and South America

OF NOTE

Other species of *Paragonimus* are also infectious for humans.

DIAGRAM 4–6. *Schistosoma* spp. (blood flukes)

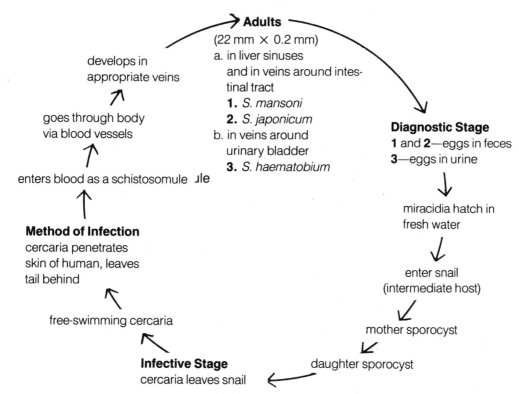

METHOD OF DIAGNOSIS

S. mansoni and *S. japonicum*—recovery of eggs in feces or rectal biopsy. *S. haematobium*—recovery of eggs in concentrated urine. Travel history, clinical symptoms and signs; serology: ELISA.

S. mansoni **egg**

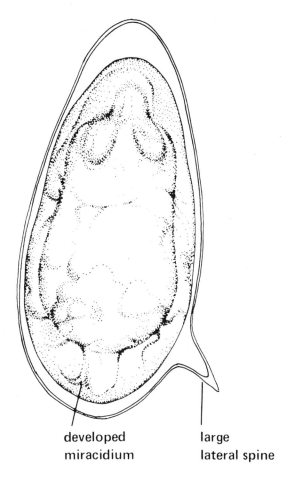

developed
miracidium

large
lateral spine

180µm × 80µm

S. haematobium **egg**

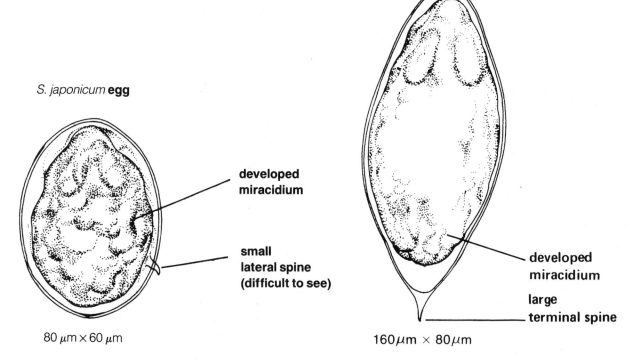

S. japonicum **egg**

developed
miracidium

small
lateral spine
(difficult to see)

80 µm × 60 µm

developed
miracidium

large
terminal spine

160µm × 80µm

DISEASE NAMES

Schistosomiasis, bilharziasis, swamp fever

MAJOR PATHOLOGY AND SYMPTOMS

1. First reaction is dermatitis.
2. Acute phase of first infection resembles typhoid fever symptoms, including fever, cough, myalgias, malaise, and hepatosplenomegaly.
3. Cirrhosis of the liver, bloody diarrhea, bowel obstruction, hypertension, and toxic reactions owing to granulomas around eggs in liver, urinary bladder, central nervous system, and other tissues.
4. Most chronic cases are asymptomatic in endemic areas. Brown hematin pigment (identical to malaria pigment) present in phagocytic cells.

TREATMENT

Praziquantel

DISTRIBUTION

S. mansoni—Africa, South and Central America, foci in the Carribean, West Indies
S. haematobium—Africa, Middle East
S. japonicum—Far East

OF NOTE

1. Schistosomiasis ranks second (behind malaria) as a cause of serious worldwide morbidity and mortality and is spreading and increasing because of recent new water-control projects which provided increased snail breeding areas.
2. *S. haematobium* has a clinical correlation with a bladder carcinoma.
3. Repeated infection with human or avian cercariae may induce allergic dermatitis (swimmer's itch) at freshwater swimming resorts. Occurs in North America.
4. Persistent Salmonella infection may be associated with *S. mansoni* and *S. japonicum*.

TABLE 4–3. Digenea

Scientific and Common Name	Epidemiology	Disease Producing Form and Its Location in Host	How Infection Occurs	Major Disease Manifestations, Diagnostic Stage, and Specimen of Choice
Fasciolopsis buski (large intestinal fluke)	Far East	Adults live in small intestine	Ingestion of encysted metacercariae on raw vegetation	Edema, eosinophilia, diarrhea, malabsorption, and even death in heavy infection Diagnosis: eggs in feces.

TABLE 4–3. *Continued*

Scientific and Common Name	Epidemiology	Disease Producing Form and Its Location in Host	How Infection Occurs	Major Disease Manifestations, Diagnostic Stage, and Specimen of Choice
Fasciola hepatica (sheep liver fluke) (zoonosis)	Worldwide (in sheep- and cattle-raising areas) Man (accidental host) Sheep (natural host)	Adults live in bile ducts	Ingestion of encysted metacercariae on raw vegetation	Traumatic tissue damage and irritation to the liver and bile ducts Jaundice and eosinophilia can occur Diagnosis: eggs in feces
Clonorchis sinensis (Oriental or Chinese liver fluke)	Far East	Adults live in bile ducts	Ingestion of encysted metacercariae in uncooked fish	Jaundice and eosinophilia in acute phase; long-term heavy infections lead to functional impairment of liver Diagnosis: eggs in feces
Paragonimus westermani (Oriental lung fluke)	Far East, India, and parts of Africa	Adults live encysted in lung	Ingestion of encysted metacercariae in uncooked crab or crayfish	Chronic fibrotic disease resembling tuberculosis—cough with blood-tinged sputum Diagnosis: eggs in sputum or feces
Heterophyes heterophyes; Metagonimus yokogawai (the heterophyids)	Far East	Adults live in small intestine	Ingestion of encysted metacercariae in uncooked fish	No intestinal symptoms unless very heavy infection Diagnosis: eggs in feces
Schistosoma mansoni (Manson's blood fluke; bilharzia; swamp fever)	Africa, Middle East, and South America	Adult in venules of the colon (eggs trapped in liver and other tissues)	Fork-tailed cercariae burrow into the capillary bed of feet, legs, or arms	Granuloma formation around eggs (i.e., in liver, intestine, and bladder)

TABLE 4–3. *Continued*

Scientific and Common Name	Epidemiology	Disease Producing Form and Its Location in Host	How Infection Occurs	Major Disease Manifestations, Diagnostic Stage, and Specimen of Choice
				Toxic and allergic reactions
				Diagnosis: eggs in feces
Schistosoma japonicum (Oriental blood fluke)	Far East	As above	As above	As above, but symptoms are more severe due to greater egg production
				Diagnosis: eggs in feces
Schistosoma haematobium (bladder fluke)	Africa, Middle East, and Portugal	Adults in venules of bladder and rectum Eggs caught in tissues	As above	Bladder colic with blood, and pus Systemic symptoms are mild Has been associated with cancer of the bladder Diagnosis: eggs in urine
Swimmer's itch (zoonosis)	Worldwide	Cercariae of schistosomes that usually parasitize mammals and birds enter human skin	Fork-tailed cercariae burrow into skin of human in water	Allergic dermal response to repeated penetration (Schistosomes do *not* develop to adults)

Be sure to examine Color Plates 53 to 71.

You have now completed the section on *Digenea*. After reviewing this material with the aid of your learning objectives, proceed to the post-test.

BIBLIOGRAPHY

ANSARI, N (ED): *Epidemiology and Control of Schistosomiasis (Bilharziasis)* S. Karger, Basel, and University Park Press, Baltimore, 1973.

HADDEN, JW AND PASCARELLI, EF: *Diagnosis and treatment of human fascioliasis.* JAMA 202:149, 1967.

HEALY, GR: *Trematodes transmitted to man by fish, frogs, and crustacea.* J Wildlife Dis 6:255, 1970.

HOW, PC: *The relationship between primary carcinoma of the liver and infestation with Clonorchis sinensis.* J Pathol Bacteriol 72:239, 1965.

VIRANUVATTI, V AND STITNIMANKARN, T: *Liver fluke infection and infestation in Southeast Asia.* Prog Liver Dis 4:537, 1972.

WARREN, KS: *The pathology of schistosome infections.* Helm Abstr Ser A 42:591, 1973.

WARREN, KS, AND MAHMOUD, AAF: *Algorithms in the diagnosis and management of exotic diseases. I. Schistosomiasis.* J Infect Dis 131:614, 1975.

YOKOGAWA, J: *Paragonimus and paragonimiasis.* IN DAWES B (ED): *Advances in Parasitology.* Academic Press, New York, 1969.

POST-TEST

1. Arrange these terms in sequence to describe the chronologic sequence of the life cycle of an intestinal trematode. (**10 points**)

   ___ egg   ___ metacercaria   ___ miracidium   ___ redia
   ___ adult   ___ sporocyst   ___ cercaria

2. You have decided to move to the Great Lakes area in the United States to become a sheep herder. You will be a hermit, living a completely self-sustained life by the edge of a lake with your sheepdog and your sheep. Which of the following set of platyhelminthes are you most likely to contract? Why did you reject each of the other answer sets? (**50 points**)

   a. *Taenia solium, Fasciola hepatica, Paragonimus westermani*
   b. *Schistosoma mansoni, Echinococcus granulosis, Clonorchis sinensis*
   c. *Fasciolopsis buski, Diphyllobothrium latum, Schistosoma japonicum*
   d. *Fasciola hepatica, Echinococcus granulosus, Diphyllobothrium latum*
   e. *Heterophyes heterophyes, Hymenolepis nana, Diphylidium caninum*

3. (**15 points**)

   a. Give the scientific and common name for each parasite represented below by the diagnostic stage.
   b. State the method of human infection by each parasite represented.

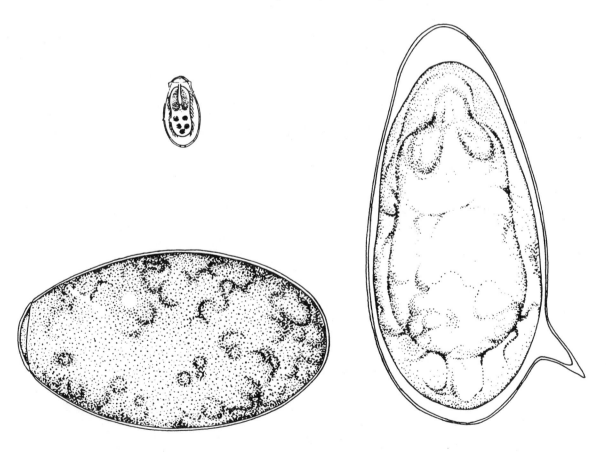

4. Why are methods of control of infection for the blood flukes different from those for the intestinal flukes? (**25 points**)

5

PROTOZOA

LEARNING OBJECTIVES

Upon completion of this chapter and its supplementary color plates as described, the student will be able to

1. state the general characteristics of each class of protozoa.
2. define terminology specific for protozoa.
3. state the recommended methods of diagnosis of protozoal infections.
4. state any vector or intermediate host involved in the transmission of specific protozoal diseases.
5. describe graphically the general life cycles for the protozoa in each class.
6. state the type of pathology caused by infection with protozoa.
7. state the scientific and common names of protozoa that parasitize humans.
8. identify accidental protozoal infections of humans that are of medical importance.
9. identify the type of specimen that would most likely contain the diagnostic stages of each pathogenic protozoan.
10. discriminate between cyst and trophozoite stages of protozoa, on the basis of both the morphologic criteria and the infectivity of various genera.
11. discriminate between pathogenic and nonpathogenic amebae on the basis of morphologic criteria.
12. differentiate species of *Plasmodium* or *Trypanosoma* by morphology and/or symptomatic criteria.
13. discuss the medical importance of accurate identification of protozoa in humans.
14. discuss the importance of protozoal zoonoses.
15. discuss how the development of genetic resistance to chemicals has an impact on protozoal diseases, such as malaria.
16. given an illustration or photograph (or an actual specimen, given sufficient laboratory experience), identify diagnostic stages of protozoa.
17. differentiate the diagnosis of protozoa and helminths.
18. compare and contrast life cycles of protozoa and helminths.
19. predict the effects of immunosuppression on patients harboring various protozoal or nematode parasites.

The subkingdom *Protozoa* includes eukaryotic unicellular animals. The various life functions are carried out by the specialized intracellular structures known as organelles. Each group of protozoa exhibits morphologic differentiation by which it can be identified.

Most protozoa multiply by binary fission. However, certain groups have more specialized modes of reproduction which will be individually discussed.

Each species of parasitic protozoa is frequently confined to one or a few host species. At least 27 species of protozoa parasitize humans, and many of these parasitic species are widely distributed throughout the world. Other vertebrates also harbor protozoan parasites, frequently without clinical signs. Parasites that have had a long co-evolution with their host species (including parasitic protozoa) have evolved adaptations that permit evasion of the host's immune recognition and response systems. It is not uncommon that accidental infection of the abnormal human host with protozoa from normal reservoir hosts causes the most serious human disease. African sleeping sickness is such an example.

There are two major methods of transmission of protozoal infection: through ingestion of the infective stage of the protozoa or by transmission via an arthropod vector. This is specific for each species.

The following groups will be considered:

1. Amebae that move by means of pseudopods
2. Protozoa that possess one to several flagella
3. Protozoa that move by means of many cilia on the cell surface
4. Protozoa that do not exhibit any obvious mode of mobility (this group uses sexual reproduction during the life cycle)

Each group will be listed in separate tables preceding the general discussion of each class of organisms. You should review the glossary before studying the rest of the chapter.

GLOSSARY

PROTOZOA. A subkingdom consisting of unicellular eukaryotic animals.

accolé. On the outer edge.

amastigote. A small, ovoid, nonflagellated form of the kinetoplastid flagellata. Notable structures include a mitochondrial kinetoplast and a large nucleus. Also called L. D. body or leishmanial form.

Apicomplexa. A phylum containing animals whose life cycle includes feeding stages (trophozoites), asexual multiplication (schizogony), and sexual multiplication (gametogony and sporogony).

atria (sing. **atrium**). An opening. In a human, refers to the mouth, vagina, and urethra.

axoneme. The intracellular portion of the flagellum.

axostyle. The axial rod functioning as a support in flagellates.

blepharoplast. The basal body origin of flagella which supports the undulating membrane in kinetoplastid flagellates.

bradyzoites. Slowly multiplying intracellular trophozoites of *Toxoplasma gondii*; form cysts in immune hosts.

carrier. A host harboring and disseminating a parasite but exhibiting no clinical signs or symptoms.

chromatin. Basophilic nuclear DNA.

chromatoidal body (or **bar**). A rod-shaped structure of condensed RNA material within the cytoplasm of some ameba cysts.

cilia. Hairlike processes attached to a free surface of a cell; functions for motility through fluids at the surface of the cell.

Ciliophora. A phylum containing animals that move by means of cilia and that have two dissimilar nuclei.

commensal. The association of two different species of organisms in which one partner is benefited and the other is neither benefited nor injured.

costa. A thin, firm, rodlike structure running along the base of the undulating membrane of certain flagellates.

cryptozoite. The stage of *Plasmodium* spp. that develops in liver cells from the inoculated sporozoites. Also called the exoerythrocytic stage or tissue stage.

cutaneous. Pertaining to the skin.

cyst. The immotile stage protected by a cyst wall formed by the parasite. In this stage, the protozoan is readily transmitted to a new host.

cytostome. The rudimentary mouth.

dysentery. A disorder marked by bloody diarrhea and/or mucus in feces.

ectoplasm. The gelatinous material beneath the cell membrane.

endoplasm. The fluid inner material of a cell.

endosome. The small mass of chromatin within the nucleus, comparable to a nucleolus of metazoan cells (also termed **karyosome**).

epimastigote. A flattened, spindle-shaped, flagellated form seen primarily in the gut (e.g., in the reduviid bug) or salivary glands (e.g., in the tsetse fly) of the vectors in the life cycle of trypanosomes; it has an undulating membrane that extends from the flagellum (attached along the anterior half of the organism) to the small kinetoplast located just anteriorly to the larger nucleus located at the midpoint of the organism.

excystation. Transformation from a cyst to a trophozoite after the cystic form has been swallowed by the host.

exflagellation. The process whereby a sporozoan microgametocyte releases haploid flagellated microgametes that can fertilize the macrogamete and thus form a diploid zygote (öokinete).

flagellum (pl. flagella). An extension of ectoplasm which provides locomotion; resembles a tail which moves with a whiplike motion.

fomite. An object that can adsorb and harbor organisms and can cause human infection by direct contact (e.g., wood or cloth).

gamete. A mature sex cell.

gametocyte. A sex cell that can produce gametes.

gametogony. The phase of the development cycle of the malaria and coccidial parasite in the human in which male and female gametocytes are formed.

hypnozoite. A long-surviving modified liver schizont of *P. vivax* which is the source of relapsing infections in this species.

karyosome. See **endosome**.

kinetoplast. An accessory body found in many protozoa, especially in the family *Trypanosomatidae*; consisting of a large mitochondrion next to the basal granule **(blepharoplast)** of the anterior or undulating membrane flagellum. Contains mitochondrial DNA.

L. D. body (Leishman-Donovan body). Each of the small ovoid amastigote forms found in tissue macrophages of the liver and spleen in patients with *Leishmania donovani* infection.

Mastigophora. A subphylum containing organisms that move by means of one or more flagella.

merogony. Asexual multiplication in coccidian life cycle. Usually occurs in intestinal epithelium.

merozoite. One of the trophozoites released from human red blood cells or liver cells at maturation of the asexual cycle of malaria.

öocyst. The encysted form of the ookinete which occurs on the stomach wall of *Anopheles* spp. mosquitoes infected with malaria.

öokinete. The motile zygote of *Plasmodium* spp.; formed by microgamete (male) fertilization of a macrogamete (female). The ookinete encysts (see oocyst).

paroxysm. The fever-chills syndrome in malaria. Spiking fever corresponds to the release of merozoites and toxic materials from the parasitized red blood cell (RBC), and shaking chills occur during schizont development. Occurs in malaria cyclically every 36 to 72 hours, depending on the species.

patent. Apparent or evident.

promastigote. A body similar to the epimastigote form except that the kinetoplast is located at the anterior end of the organism, and therefore has no undulating membrane. This form is seen in the midgut and pharynx of vectors in the life cycle of the leishmania parasites and will be the form seen in culture media *in vitro*.

pseudopod. A protoplasmic extension of the trophozoites of amebae that allows them to move and to engulf food.

pseudocyst. A cystlike structure formed by the host during an acute infection with *Tox-*

oplasma gondii. The cyst is filled with tachyzoites in normal hosts; may occur in brain or other tissues. Latent source of infection which may become active if immunosuppression occurs.

Sarcodina. A subphylum containing amebae that move by means of pseudopodia.

schizogony (merogony). Asexual multiplication of *Apicomplexa;* multiple intracellular nuclear division precedes cytoplasmic division.

schizont. The developed stage of asexual division of the *Sporozoa* trophozoite (e.g., *Plasmodium* spp. in a human red blood cell, *Isospora belli* in the intestinal wall).

sporocyst. The fertilized öocyst in which the sporozoites of *Plasmodium* have developed.

sporogony. Sexual reproduction of *Apicomplexa.* Production of spores and sporozoites.

sporozoite. The form of *Plasmodium* that develops inside the sporocyst, invades the salivary glands of the mosquito, and is transmitted to humans.

subpatent. Not evident, subclinical.

tachyzoites. Rapidly growing intracellular trophozoites of *Toxoplasma gondii.*

trophozoite. The motile stage of protozoan which feeds, multiplies, and maintains the colony within the host.

trypomastigote. A body similar to the epimastigote form except that the kinetoplast is located at the posterior end of the organism and the undulating membrane extends along the entire body from the flagellum (anterior end) to the posterior end at the blepharoplast. This form is seen in the blood of humans with trypanosomiasis and as the infective stage in the insect vectors.

undulating membrane. A protoplasmic membrane with a flagellar rim extending out like a fin along the outer edge of the body of certain protozoa; it moves in a wavelike pattern.

xenodiagnosis. Infections with *Trypanosoma cruzi* may be diagnosed by allowing an uninfected *Triatoma* bug to feed on the patient (the bite is painless); the insect's feces are later examined for parasites (trypanosome forms).

zygote. The fertilized cell resulting from the union of male and female gametes.

CLASS LOBOSEA

These amebae in the order Amoebida (Table 5–1), which are parasites of humans, can be found worldwide. The motile, reproducing feeding stage (the **trophozoite**) lives most commonly in the lower gastrointestinal tract. Many of these amebae can form a nonfeeding, nonmotile **cyst** stage, which is the stage that is infective for man. Transmission of amebae is generally by ingestion of cysts in fecally contaminated food or water. When cysts are swallowed and pass to the lower intestine, they **excyst** and begin to multiply as feeding **trophozoites.**

The structure of the nucleus is quite different for each genus of ameba, and identification of nuclear structure aids in diagnosis. A permanent stain such as the Trichrome stain used on a thin fixed fecal smear is particularly helpful in identifying nuclear structures and is highly recommended as a routine procedure in a diagnostic laboratory. Other diagnostic features include size, cytoplasmic inclusions, and type of motility exhibited by the **pseudopods** formed by trophozoites in a wet-mount preparation. In the cyst stage, nuclear structure, the size and shape of the cyst, the number of nuclei, and other inclusion bodies present are diagnostic features.

Entamoeba histolytica is the major pathogen in this group and is the cause of amebic dysentery in humans. It can occur in other primates, dogs, cats, and rats. All other amebae seen in feces are considered to be nonpathogenic **commensals.** It is important, however, that each species be correctly identified to insure proper therapy, if needed, and to avoid unnecessary treatment owing to misdiagnosis.

The nucleus of *Entamoeba histolytica* has a small central **karyosome (endosome)** and uniform peripheral chromatin granules lining the nuclear membrane. *E. histolytica*

TABLE 5–1. Amebae

Order	Scientific Name	Common Name
Amoebida	*Entamoeba histolytica* (en'tuh-mee'buh/his-toe-lit'i-kuh)	Amebic dysentery
Amoebida	*Entamoeba hartmanni* (en'tuh-mee'buh/hart-man'nee)	Small race of *E. histolytica*
Amoebida	*Entamoeba coli* (en'tuh-mee'buh/ko'lye)	Commensal
Amoebida	*Endolimax nana* (en'doe-lye'macks/nay'nuh)	Commensal
Amoebida	*Iodamoeba bütschlii* (eye-o'duh-mee'buh/bootch'lee-eye)	Commensal
Amoebida	*Acanthamoeba* spp. (ay-kanth'uh-mee'buh)	None
Schizopyrenida	*Naegleria fowleri* (nay'gleer-ee'uh fow-ler'i)	Primary amebic meningoencephalitis

invades the intestinal wall and multiplies in the mucosal tissue. In the cytoplasm of the trophozoite, one can frequently see ingested red blood cells; the trophozoite voraciously feeds on these red blood cells when it is invasive. The red blood cells can appear either whole or partially digested. These blood cells will not be seen in the trophozoite of any other ameba, and their presence helps in differential diagnosis. The trophozoite of *E. histolytica* extends thin pseudopods and exhibits active, progressive motility in a wet mount.

The cyst of *E. histolytica* contains one, two, or four nuclei: nuclear divisions accompany cyst maturation. The nuclear structure, as seen in stained cysts or in trophozoites, is the same.

The cyst of the pathogenic *E. histolytica* is round and is 10 to 20 μm in size. It may also contain cigar-shaped **chromatoidal bars**. There is a small race of *E. histolytica* identified as *Entamoeba hartmanni*, which forms cysts of less than 10 μm. *E. hartmanni* is nonpathogenic. A calibrated ocular micrometer is required to measure cyst diameters. Pathology caused by *E. histolytica* includes flask-shaped ulcerations of the intestinal wall and bloody dysentery. If amebae penetrate the intestinal wall and spread via blood, ulceration may occur in the liver, lungs, brain, or other tissues. This can be fatal. Prevalence is very high in the subtropics and tropics (over 50 percent), and focal epidemics can occur anywhere. Prevalence in the U.S. and Europe is around 5 percent, with most being **carriers.**

Entamoeba coli (a nonpathogenic commensal) is most commonly confused with *E. histolytica*. The nucleus of *E. coli* differs from *E. histolytica*; it has a large eccentric karyosome and irregular peripheral chromatin clumping along the nuclear membrane. The trophozoite exhibits granular cytoplasm and ingested bacteria, but not red blood cells. Motility is sluggish. The cyst stage often has up to eight nuclei of characteristic structure rather than a maximum of four as in *E. histolytica*. Chromatoidal bars, if present, have pointed rather than rounded ends.

Cysts of amebae may have varying numbers of nuclei depending on their stage of development; therefore, it is critical to look at nuclear structure as well as numbers for identification. Additionally, *Dientamoeba fragilis* (a flagellate) may occasionally have more or less than two nuclei in the trophozoite stage and could therefore be confused with developing cysts of *Endolimax nana* or other ameba.

Several species of free-living amebae may become opportunistic parasites of humans. These organisms are found in fresh or salt water, moist soil, and decaying vegetation. In most instances, no disease is produced by these organisms, but in a few cases, severe consequences result. The notable potential pathogens are *Naegleria fowleri* and, less commonly, *Acanthamoeba* spp. *Naegleria* is actually an ameboflagelelate, because in the free-living state, it alternates from an ameboid phase to a form possessing two flagella. Only the ameboid phase is found in host tissues.

The disease caused by *N. fowleri* occurs most often during the summer months. The parasite gains entry through the nasal mucosa when the host is diving and swimming in ponds or small lakes which are inhabited by the parasite. This parasite tolerates chlorinated water and has even been found in an indoor swimming pool. Furthermore, infections have been acquired by drinking unfiltered, chlorinated tapwater. Upon infection, the clinical symptoms are very dramatic, and the disease runs a very rapid and usually fatal course. Symptoms begin with a headache, fever, nausea, and vomiting within 1 or 2 days. Typical symptoms of meningoencephalitis follow, leading to irrational behavior, coma, and death. The clinical course rarely lasts more than 6 days.

Diagnosis is often made on autopsy; however, a purulent spinal fluid containing high numbers of neutrophils (200 to 20,000/μl) without bacteria should add amebic meningoencephalitis to the differential diagnosis. Motile amebae may be noted in unstained preparations. Treatment is usually unsuccessful; however, amphotericin B and sulfadiazine have been effective in a very few cases. Early diagnosis and immediate treatment is crucial.

Acanthamoeba spp. cause a more chronic form of meningoencephalitis. Infected patients frequently have compromised immunologic systems. Onset of symptoms is slow, usually 10 days or more. Chronic granulomatous lesions in brain tissue may contain both trophozoites and cysts. These parasites have been found in lungs, nasal passages, eyes, ears, skin lesions, and the vagina. Infection of the eyes (keratitis) seems to be found more frequently in patients who wear soft contact lenses.

Cysts of *Acanthamoeba* spp., like *Naegleria* spp., are also resistant to chlorination and drying. The parasite may be transported by water and possibly through air.

DIAGRAM 5–1. *Entamoeba histolytica* (ameba)

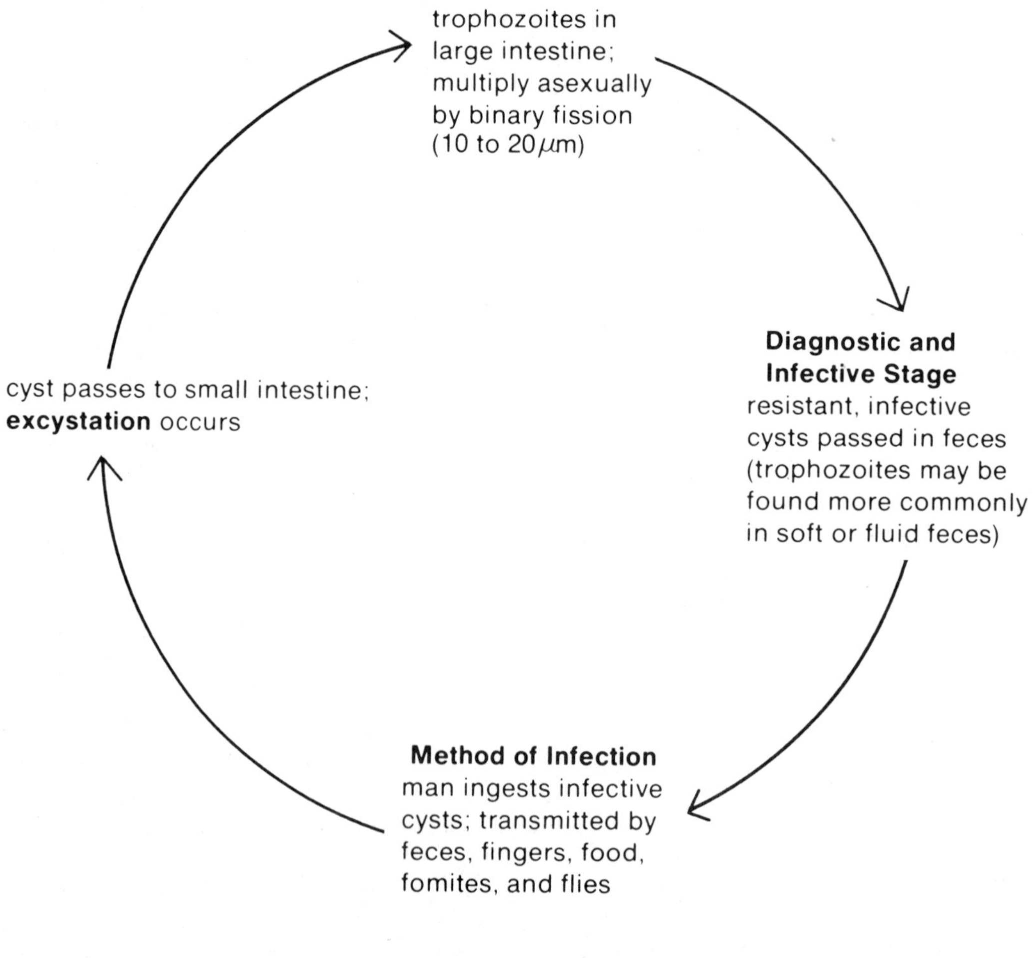

trophozoites in large intestine; multiply asexually by binary fission (10 to 20 μm)

Diagnostic and Infective Stage
resistant, infective cysts passed in feces (trophozoites may be found more commonly in soft or fluid feces)

cyst passes to small intestine; **excystation** occurs

Method of Infection
man ingests infective cysts; transmitted by feces, fingers, food, fomites, and flies

METHOD OF DIAGNOSIS

Recovery and identification of trophozoites or cysts in feces or intestinal mucosa. Serology: indirect hemagglutination for liver infection.

DIAGNOSTIC STAGE

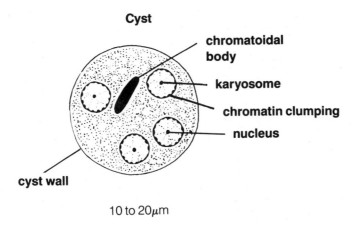

Cyst

chromatoidal body

karyosome

chromatin clumping

nucleus

cyst wall

10 to 20μm

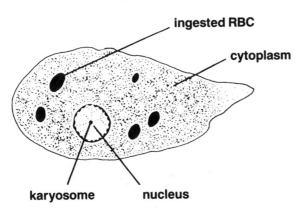

Trophozoite

ingested RBC

cytoplasm

karyosome   nucleus

10 to 20 μm

DISEASE NAMES

Amebiasis, amebic dysentery, amebic hepatitis (if liver is involved)

MAJOR PATHOLOGY AND SYMPTOMS

May be asymptomatic or exhibit vague abdominal discomfort, malaise, diarrhea alternating with constipation, or if acute, bloody dysentery and fever. Invades intestinal submucosa via lytic enzymes; lateral extension leads to typical flask-shaped lesions. In amebic hepatitis there is an enlarged liver, fever, chills, and leukocytosis.

TREATMENT

Depends on location of infection: iodoquinol, diloxamide, paromomycin, metronida-zole, dehydroemetine, and combinations (see *Medical Letter* items in Bibliography on page 159).

DISTRIBUTION

Worldwide

OF NOTE

1. Chronic infection may last for years.
2. Must be differentiated from ulcerative colitis, carcinoma, other intestinal para-sites, and diverticulitis, and also must differentiate hepatic form from hepatitis, hydatid cyst, various gall bladder problems, cancer, or lung disease.
3. Ameba can invade lungs, brain, skin, and so forth. Hepatic amebiasis is the most common and most grave complication. Usually there is only a single abscess in the right lobe of the liver.

Comparative Morphology of Intestinal Amebae

Cyst   **Trophozoite**

Entamoeba histolytica

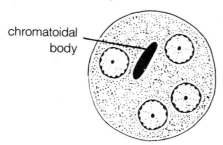

chromatoidal body

Red blood cells being digested

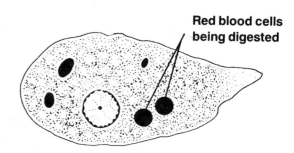

diameter over 10 μm, up to 4 nuclei,
central karyosome, even nuclear chromatin at edges

Cyst   **Trophozoite**

Entamoeba hartmanni

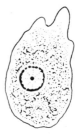

diameter less than 10 μm

Cyst

Trophozoite

Entamoeba coli

bacteria

**chromatoidal
body**

diameter over 10 μm, up to 8 nucleii,
eccentric karyosome, irregular nuclear chromatin

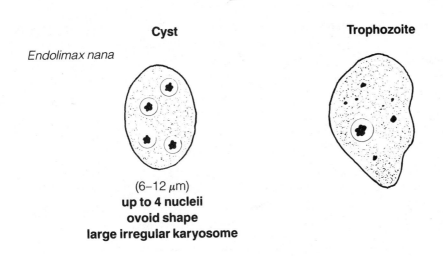

Cyst

Trophozoite

Endolimax nana

(6–12 μm)
**up to 4 nucleii
ovoid shape
large irregular karyosome**

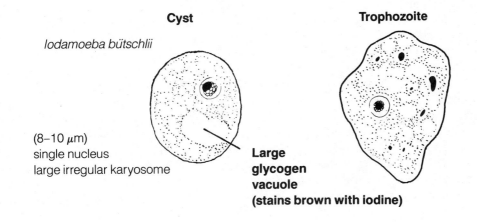

Cyst

Trophozoite

Iodamoeba bütschlii

(8–10 μm)
single nucleus
large irregular karyosome

**Large
glycogen
vacuole
(stains brown with iodine)**

SUPERCLASS MASTIGOPHORA

Flagellates in the class *Zoomastigophorea* include the pathogenic protozoa that inhabit the gastrointestinal tract, **atria,** blood stream, or tissues of humans. The parasites considered in this group are listed in Table 5–2. The pathogenic intestinal flagellates include genera in only two of the species, *Giardia lamblia* and *Dientamoeba fragilis*. Two common nonpathogenic species found in the intestinal tract include *Chilomastix mesnili* and *Trichomonas hominis*. These organisms must be differentiated from pathogens to avoid misdiagnosis and mistreatment. There is only one pathogenic atrial protozoan—*Trichomonas vaginalis*—that inhabits the vagina and urethra. In the order *Kinetoplastida*, there

TABLE 5–2. Flagellates

Order	Scientific Name	Common Name
Diplomonadida	*Giardia lamblia* (gee'are-dee'uh/lamb-blee'uh)	traveler's diarrhea
Trichomonadida	*Dientamoeba fragilis* (dye-en'tuh-mee'buh/fradj"i-lis)	Dientamoeba
Trichomonadida	*Trichomonas vaginalis* (trick"o-mo'nas/vadj-i-nay'lis)	trich
Kinetoplastida	*Trypanosoma rhodesiense* (trip-an"o-so"muh/ro-dee"zee-en'see)	East African sleeping sickness
Kinetoplastida	*Trypanosoma gambiense* (trip-an"o-so'muh/gam-bee-en'see)	West African sleeping sickness
Kinetoplastida	*Trypanosoma cruzi* (trip-an'o-so'muh/kroo'zye)	Chagas' disease
Kinetoplastida	*Leishmania tropica* (leesh-may'nee-uh/trop'i-kuh)	Oriental sore
Kinetoplastida	*Leishmania braziliensis* (leesh-may'nee-uh/bra-zil"i-en'sis)	New World leishmaniasis
Kinetoplastida	*Leishmania donovani* (leesh-may'nee-uh/don"o-vay'nigh)	kala-azar

are two genera that are pathogenic and multiply in the tissues of humans. These are the genus *Trypanosoma*, which has three major pathogenic species, and the genus *Leishmania*, which also has three major pathogenic species.

Giardia lamblia is the most common intestinal parasite in the United States. Of the intestinal flagellates, it is important to differentiate *Giardia lamblia* from the several nonpathogenic flagellates which can be found in the intestinal tract. The trophozoite and the cyst of two of these are illustrated on page 76. The trophozoite of *G. lamblia* (10–20 μm $\times$ 5–15 μm) is bilaterally symmetric and has two anterior nuclei and eight **flagella.** A sucking disk concavity on the ventral side is the means of attachment to the intestinal mucosa. The cysts are oval with two or four nuclei located at one end. The clustered nuclei and the central **axostyle** give the cyst the appearance of "a little old lady wearing glasses." The cytoplasm is often retracted from the cyst wall, leaving a clear space under the wall. This parasite has frequently been associated with traveler's diarrhea, and both trophozoites and cysts can be found in the diarrheic feces along with unusual amounts of mucus. These are not tissue invaders; however, prolonged heavy infection may result in malabsorption by the intestinal mucosa. Transmission is by ingestion of the cyst stage in fecally contaminated water or food.

Dientamoeba fragilis also has been associated with cases of diarrhea. *D. fragilis* lives in the cecum and colon and does not form cysts; the method of transmission is uncertain. The trophozoite has two nuclei connected by a division spindle filament. *D. fragilis* has no observable flagella but is classified as a trichomonad even though it moves by means of pseudopodia rather than flagella when seen in feces. The trophozoite is 6–20 μm and exhibits sluggish nondirectional motility.

Trichomonas vaginalis multiplies in the genitourinary atrium of both males and females. Usually only females exhibit symptoms, and males serve as asymptomatic **carriers.** Transmission of *T. vaginalis* is generally by sexual intercourse. Trichomonad species do not form cysts. Motile *T. vaginalis* trophozoites may be identified in a fresh urine or in a urethral or vaginal smear by its characteristic structure. There is a large anterior nucleus, four anterior flagella, an axostyle, and an **undulating membrane.** Even though the male is usually asymptomatic, all sex partners should be treated so that reinfection of the female partner does not recur.

In the order Kinetoplastida, the pathogenic *Trypanosoma* and *Leishmania* flagellates multiply in the blood (hemoflagellates) or tissue of humans. All species require an arthropod intermediate host. Furthermore, the hemoflagellates exhibit specific morphology in specific locations in both humans and arthropods.

In the genus *Trypanosoma*, two species, *T. rhodesiense* and *T. gambiense*, cause East and West African sleeping sickness, respectively. These diseases are transmitted by the tsetse fly intermediate host (*Glossina* ssp.). Organisms are injected when the infected fly takes a blood meal. The **trypomastigote** form can be found in a human blood smear extracellularly in the plasma or in tissues such as lymph node biopsies or in the central nervous system late in the disease.

The species *Trypanosoma cruzi,* primarily found in Central and South America, causes a debilitating condition known as Chagas' disease. *T. cruzi* is transmitted by the *Triatoma* bug intermediate host. When the *Triatoma* takes a blood meal, infective organisms are deposited on the skin in the feces of the bug and are rubbed into the wound when the itching bite site is scratched. *T. cruzi* organisms multiply in macrophages of the reticuloendothelial system and are found multiplying in tissues such as heart as the **amastigote** form. However, trypomastigote and **epimastigote** forms may be found in the blood stream early during the infection. Chagas' disease can result in enlarged heart, esophagus, and colon, and eventually in death, if untreated. In children, an acute fatal disease course is not uncommon.

In the genus *Leishmania*, there are four pathogenic "species complexes" with subspecies in each complex: *L. tropica* (Old World), *L. mexicana* (New World), *L. braziliensis,* and *L. donovani.* Speciation has traditionally been based on clinical symptomology, geographic location, and case history. All *Leishmania* species are transmitted by the sand fly intermediate host *Phlebotomus* spp. The bite of an infected sand fly results initially in a self-healing lesion of the skin at the bite site, which may last up to a year and may be a wet or dry ulcer, depending on the species. Amastigote forms can be found multiplying intracellularly in local macrophages of the lesion. *L. tropica* and *L. mexicana* cause cutaneous, spontaneously healing ulcers, although some subspecies of *L. mexicana* spread to cause disfiguring diffuse cutaneous leishmaniasis (DCL). *L. braziliensis* affects the mucosa of the nasopharynx and mouth. Additionally, *Leishmania braziliensis* can become **subpatent** and can flare up years later, resulting in erosion of cartilage in the nose and ears.

Unlike the others, *L. donovani* does not stay localized in the skin lesion and will spread to the viscera, multiplying in macrophages of all internal organs, and eventually causes death if the patient is untreated. In tissue sections (e.g., liver or spleen), *L. donovani* can be seen as intracellular multiplying amastigote forms **(L.D. bodies)**. All species of Leishmania that infect humans are zoonoses; the usual host is a vertebrate such as a dog, fox, or rodent.

DIAGRAM 5–2. *Giardia lamblia* (flagellate)

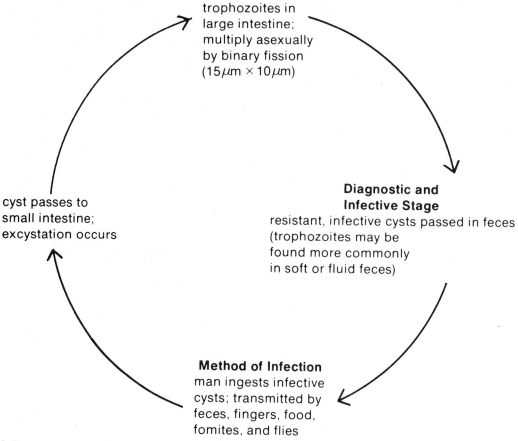

trophozoites in
large intestine;
multiply asexually
by binary fission
($15\,\mu m \times 10\,\mu m$)

**Diagnostic and
Infective Stage**
resistant, infective cysts passed in feces
(trophozoites may be
found more commonly
in soft or fluid feces)

cyst passes to
small intestine;
excystation occurs

Method of Infection
man ingests infective
cysts; transmitted by
feces, fingers, food,
fomites, and flies

METHOD OF DIAGNOSIS

Recovery and identification of trophozoites or cysts in feces or duodenal contents.*

DIAGNOSTIC STAGE

Cyst

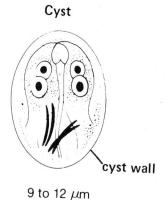

cyst wall

9 to 12 μm

Trophozoite

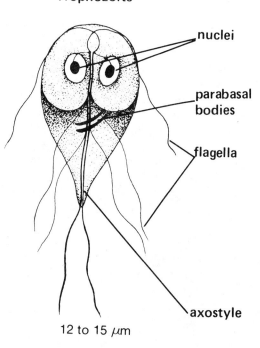

nuclei

parabasal
bodies

flagella

axostyle

12 to 15 μm

*A commercially available, orally retrievable string device (swallowed in a gelatin capsule)—Enterotest (available from "Hedeco"—Health Development Corp., East Palo Alto, CA) can be examined for the presence of trophozoites in duodenal mucus adherent on the string, which is pulled up after swallowing. It is also useful for recovering *Strongyloides stercoralis* eggs and/or larvae.

DISEASE NAMES

Giardiasis, traveler's diarrhea

MAJOR PATHOLOGY AND SYMPTOMS

Abdominal pain, foul-smelling diarrhea, foul-smelling gas, mechanical irritation of intestinal mucosa with shortening of villi and inflammatory foci; malabsorption syndrome in heavy infections. Persons with an immunoglobulin class A deficiency may be more susceptible. Stool does not contain red or white blood cells as in bacillary dysentery.

TREATMENT

1. quinacrine
2. metronidazole or furazolidone

DISTRIBUTION

Worldwide

OF NOTE

1. Recent outbreaks have been related to cross-contamination of water and sewage systems as well as to suspicion that wild animals such as beavers serve as reservoir hosts.
2. Travelers to endemic areas (such as Leningrad in the Soviet Union and some American areas as well) experience severe diarrhea upon infection, but permanent residents of the endemic areas generally do not.

DIAGRAM 5–3. *Dientamoeba fragilis* (intestinal flagellate)

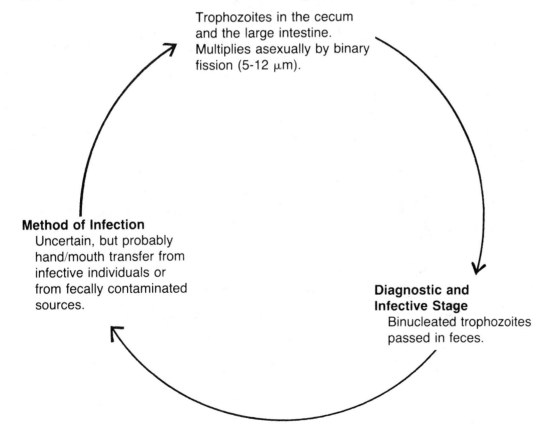

Trophozoites in the cecum and the large intestine. Multiplies asexually by binary fission (5-12 μm).

Method of Infection
Uncertain, but probably hand/mouth transfer from infective individuals or from fecally contaminated sources.

Diagnostic and Infective Stage
Binucleated trophozoites passed in feces.

METHOD OF DIAGNOSIS

Identification of trophozoites in feces (no cyst stage known)

DIAGNOSTIC STAGE

Dientamoeba fragilis   (two nuclei)

**No cyst
stage
known**

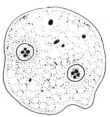

MAJOR PATHOLOGY AND SYMPTOMS

Usually asymptomatic; may be associated with diarrhea, anorexia, abdominal pain.

TREATMENT

Iodoquinol, tetracycline, or paromomycin

DISTRIBUTION

Worldwide

OF NOTE

1. A fairly high association between *Enterobius vermicularis* and *D. fragilis* infections has been noted. These findings suggest that *D. fragilis* infections may also be transmitted via pinworm eggs.
2. No cyst stage is known for this parasite.
3. Most organisms will have two nuclei. As many as 40 percent may have only one nucleus.

Nonpathogenic Intestinal Flagellates

Chilomastix mesnili

Cyst   **Trophozoite**

**clear knob on
cyst**

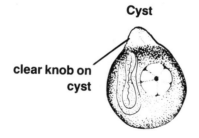

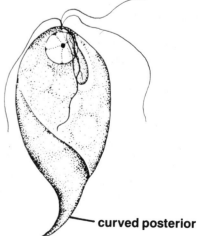

curved posterior

Trichomonas hominis

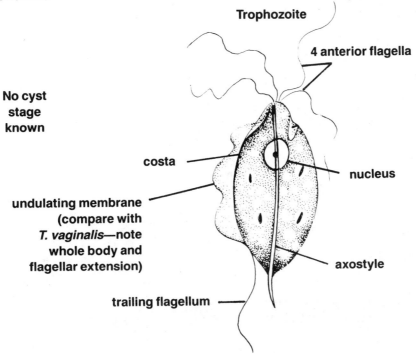

Trophozoite

4 anterior flagella

No cyst stage known

costa

nucleus

undulating membrane (compare with *T. vaginalis*—note whole body and flagellar extension)

axostyle

trailing flagellum

DIAGRAM 5–4. *Trichomonas vaginalis* (atrial flagellate)

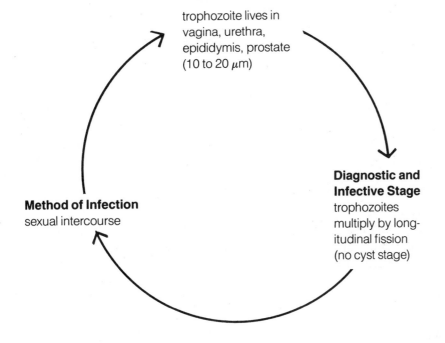

trophozoite lives in vagina, urethra, epididymis, prostate (10 to 20 μm)

Diagnostic and Infective Stage trophozoites multiply by longitudinal fission (no cyst stage)

Method of Infection sexual intercourse

METHOD OF DIAGNOSIS

Recovery and identification of motile trophozoites in a fresh urethral discharge, vaginal smear, or urine. Can be recognized in Papanicolaou stained cervical smears.

DIAGNOSTIC STAGE

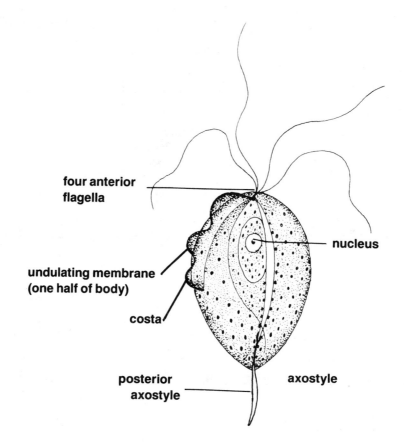

four anterior
flagella

nucleus

undulating membrane
(one half of body)

costa

posterior
axostyle

axostyle

Trophozoite (no cyst stage form)
15 μm

DISEASE NAMES

Trichomonad vaginitis, urethritis, trich

MAJOR PATHOLOGY AND SYMPTOMS

1. Female:
    a. persistent vaginal inflammation
    b. yellowish frothy foul-smelling vaginal discharge
    c. burning urination
    d. itching and irritation

2. Male: generally asymptomatic

TREATMENT

Metronidazole

DISTRIBUTION

Worldwide

DIAGRAM 5–5. *Trypanosoma rhodesiense* (East African sleeping sickness) and *Trypanosoma gambiense* (West African sleeping sickness)

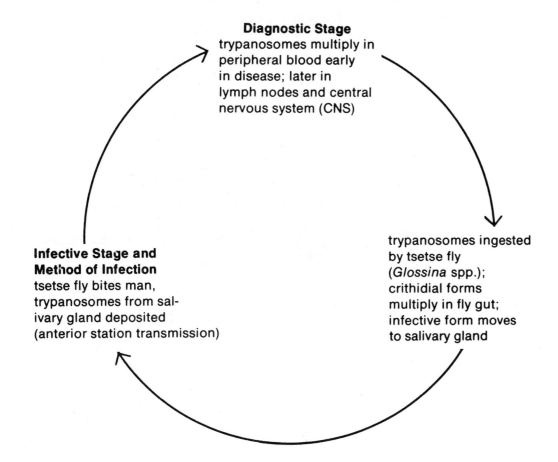

Diagnostic Stage
trypanosomes multiply in peripheral blood early in disease; later in lymph nodes and central nervous system (CNS)

trypanosomes ingested by tsetse fly (*Glossina* spp.); crithidial forms multiply in fly gut; infective form moves to salivary gland

Infective Stage and Method of Infection
tsetse fly bites man, trypanosomes from salivary gland deposited (anterior station transmission)

METHOD OF DIAGNOSIS

Examine fluid from bite site chancre or buffy coat of blood for trypomastigotes during febrile period. Thick blood smears (see page 135) increase the chance of diagnosis. Late in infection, trypomastigotes can be best found in lymph nodes or cerebrospinal fluid. Animal innoculation (mice or young rats) may be helpful.

DIAGNOSTIC STAGE

Trypomastigote form in plasma

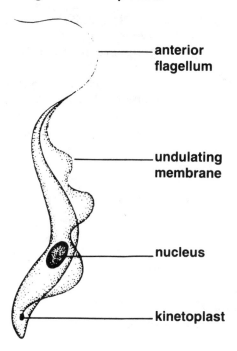

anterior
flagellum

undulating
membrane

nucleus

kinetoplast

15 to 30 μm × 1.5 to 3.5 μm

DISEASE NAME

African sleeping sickness

MAJOR PATHOLOGY AND SYMPTOMS

Pathology and symptoms for both parasites include

1. lesion of bite site (chancre) usually seen in non-Africans
2. enlarged lymph nodes, especially posterior cervical chain (Winterbottom sign)
3. fever, headache, night sweats
4. joint and muscle pain
5. central nervous system (CNS) impairment in 6 months to 1 year with *T. gambiense* but in 1 month with *T. rhodesiense*
6. lethargy and motor changes
7. coma and death; death from cardiac failure may precede CNS symptoms in *T. rhodesiense*

TREATMENT

Depends on phase of disease. Early: suramin or pentamidine; late: melarsoprol or tryparsamide, when CNS involvement has occurred.

DISTRIBUTION

Primarily Africa, as noted.

OF NOTE

1. Red blood cell autoagglutination is commonly observed in vitro.
2. High levels of immunoglobulin M (IgM) and high levels of spinal fluid proteins are characteristic.
3. IgM in spinal fluid is diagnostic.

DIAGRAM 5–6. *Trypanosoma cruzi* (Chagas' disease)

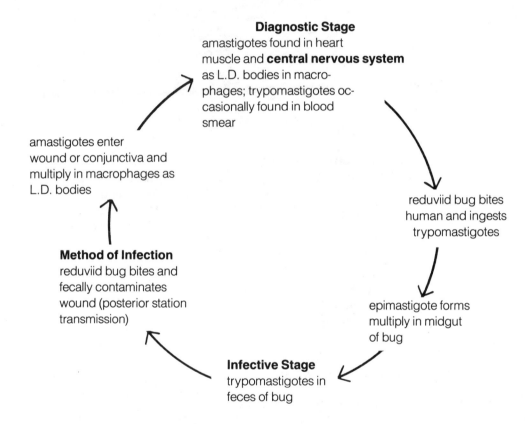

Diagnostic Stage
amastigotes found in heart muscle and **central nervous system** as L.D. bodies in macrophages; trypomastigotes occasionally found in blood smear

amastigotes enter wound or conjunctiva and multiply in macrophages as L.D. bodies

Method of Infection
reduviid bug bites and fecally contaminates wound (posterior station transmission)

reduviid bug bites human and ingests trypomastigotes

epimastigote forms multiply in midgut of bug

Infective Stage
trypomastigotes in feces of bug

METHOD OF DIAGNOSIS

1. Finding amastigotes in stained tissue scraping of skin lesion (chagoma) at bite site.
2. Identification of C-shaped trypomastigotes in blood smear during acute exacerbation.
3. **Xenodiagnosis**—allow uninfected bugs to feed on patient, then later examine bug feces for parasite.
4. Serology—Machado complement fixation test, intradermal test, or indirect hemagglutination test; EVI (endocardial, vascular, and interstitial) antibodies present.
5. L.D. bodies (amastigotes) in heart muscle postmortem.
6. Culture in diphasic Novy, MacNeal, and Nicolle (N.N.N.) medium (see page 134)

Diagnostic Stage

**Pseudocyst containing amastigote stages
in heart muscle**

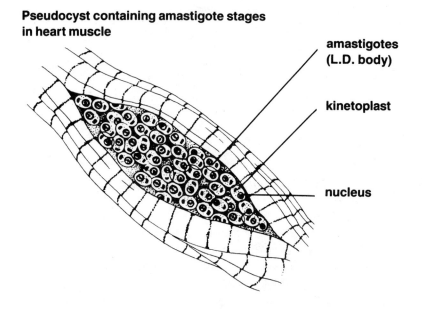

amastigotes
(L.D. body)

kinetoplast

nucleus

**C- or S-shaped trypomastigote
form in blood**

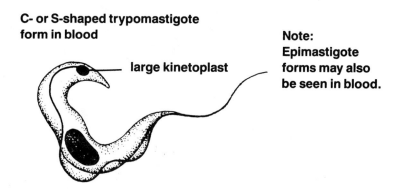

large kinetoplast

**Note:
Epimastigote
forms may also
be seen in blood.**

Disease Names

Chagas' disease, American trypanosomiasis

Major Pathology and Symptoms

1. In chronic cases, usually in adults, there may be no history of acute illness, but enlarged flabby heart may cause sudden death.
2. May be fever, weakness, enlarged spleen, liver, and lymph nodes.
3. Acute infection (most common in children) results in initial chagoma reaction at bite site with periorbital edema if bitten near the eye (Romaña's sign), cardiac ganglia destruction, megacolon, and often rapid death.

Treatment

Nifurtimox

Distribution

Mexico, Central America, and South America; cause of 30 percent of adult deaths in Brazil. Few cases in Texas and California.

Of Note

1. Many animals serve as reservoir hosts in the warmer southwestern states of North America.
2. Bugs feed at night on warm-blooded hosts, frequently on the conjunctiva of the eye.
3. *T. cruzi* can cross the placenta and cause prenatal disease.
4. Autoimmune reaction by antibodies that cross-react with endocardium, vascular structures, and interstitium of smooth muscle (EVI antibodies) may play a role in heart, colon, and esophagus dilation and atony.
5. Nonpathogenic *T. rangeli* trypomastigotes may be present in humans in Central and South America and may confuse diagnosis.

DIAGRAM 5–7. *Leishmania tropica, L. mexicana, L. braziliensis,* and *L. donovani* species complexes (Leishmaniasis)

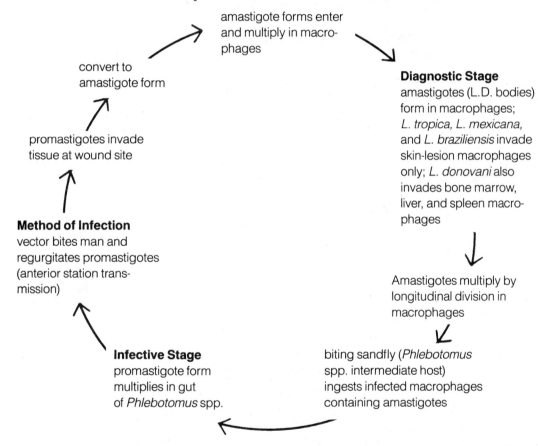

amastigote forms enter and multiply in macrophages

convert to amastigote form

promastigotes invade tissue at wound site

Method of Infection
vector bites man and regurgitates promastigotes (anterior station transmission)

Infective Stage
promastigote form multiplies in gut of *Phlebotomus* spp.

Diagnostic Stage
amastigotes (L.D. bodies) form in macrophages; *L. tropica, L. mexicana,* and *L. braziliensis* invade skin-lesion macrophages only; *L. donovani* also invades bone marrow, liver, and spleen macrophages

Amastigotes multiply by longitudinal division in macrophages

biting sandfly (*Phlebotomus* spp. intermediate host) ingests infected macrophages containing amastigotes

Method of Diagnosis

L. tropica and *L. mexicana*—identification of amastigotes in macrophages of skin lesion.
L. braziliensis—identification of amastigotes at the periphery of the lesion.
L. donovani—identification of amastigotes in early skin lesion and L.D. bodies later in reticuloendothelial system, spleen, lymph nodes, bone marrow, and liver. Also present in feces, urine, and nasal discharges. Clinical symptoms in person in endemic area presumptive; bone marrow smears helpful; striking increase in gamma globulin; serology, skin testing, culture, and animal inoculation helpful.

Diagnostic Stage

Amastigotes multiplying in tissue macrophages

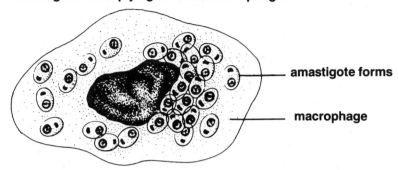

amastigote forms

macrophage

macrophage nucleus

Disease Names

L. tropica—cutaneous or Old World leishmaniasis, Oriental sore, Baghdad or Delhi boil
L. braziliensis—mucocutaneous or New World leishmaniasis, uta, espundia
L. donovani—visceral leishmaniasis, kala-azar, Dumdum fever

Major Pathology and Symptoms

The type of illness is due to immunopathology in specific tissue sites.

1. *L. tropica* complex
   Incubation period: several months. One or more self-healing ulcerated pus-filled lesions on body (indurated with macrophages); self-healing. Lesions often moist and short term in rural areas (infection by *L. major* lasting 3 to 6 months), dry and long lasting in urban areas (infection by *L. tropica*, lasting 12 to 18 months).
   Treatment: 1. antimony, 2. local heat (39° to 42°C) for 12 hours on chancre

2. *L. mexicana*
   Similar to *L. tropica*. Two subspecies may cause diffuse cutaneous leishmaniasis (DCL).
   Treatment: 1. antimony, 2. amphotericin B

3. *L. braziliensis*
   Red, itchy indurated ulcer; lesions may metastasize along lymphatics; self-healing. Disfigurement of nose and ears may occur years later from chronic mucosal ulceration. Diffuse cutaneous leishmaniasis, seen mainly in Brazil, has an absence of cell-mediated immune reactivity. Note: May be caused by *L. pifanoi*.
   Treatment: 1. antimony, 2. amphotericin B

4. *L. donovani*
   Long incubation period. Initial lesion: short-term small papules at bite site. Malarialike spiking chills and fever (double fever spike daily); sweating, diarrhea, dysentery, weight loss; splenomegaly and hepatomegaly after leishmania disseminate and multiply in visceral reticuloendothelium. Hyperplasia of tissue and organs. Progressive anemia. Causes death if untreated, often from secondary infection.
   Treatment: 1. antimony, 2. pentamidine isothionate

Distribution

L. tropica complex: Mediterranean area, southwestern Asia, central and northwest Africa, Central America and South America; recent cases in Texas (may be *L. mexicana*)
L. braziliensis: Central America and South America; highest concentration in Brazil and the Andes; rural disease

L. donovani: North Africa and east Africa, Asia, Mediterranean area, and South America; primarily in young children. India and Bangladesh; primarily in adults.

OF NOTE

1. Cutaneous lesions may appear as ulcers, as cauliflowerlike masses, or as nodules.
2. Host's genetic, nutritional, and immunologic status plays a large role in pathology.
3. A variety of animals serves as reservoir hosts (e.g., gerbils and other rodents—monkeys and dogs in the New World).
4. Vaccination against *L. tropica* is common in U.S.S.R.
5. Leishmanian skin test becomes positive in DCL and kala-azar only after cure.
6. Elevated levels of gamma globulin are present in leishmaniasis.
7. *L. tropica* generally transmitted from humans as hosts; other parasites in the complex are primarily zoonoses.

CLASS KINETOFRAGMINOPHOREA

Organisms in this class are characterized by ectoplasmic **cilia** covering the surface, two different kinds of nuclei (a large kidney-shaped macronucleus and a small micronucleus), and other well-developed organelles such as an oral **cytostome.** Ciliates multiply asexually by binary fission and also have sexual reproduction by conjugation with exchange of micronuclei.

Balantidium coli (bal'an-tid'ee-um/ko'lye) is the largest parasitic protozoan (60 μm × 40 μm) and is the only ciliate that is pathogenic for humans. *B. coli* causes dysentery in severe intestinal infections and can be found in feces in either the trophozoite or cyst state. It is probable that human infections are directly acquired through ingestion of cysts in fecally contaminated food or water.

This parasite is a tissue invader and produces intestinal lesions along the submucosa. There are also reports of vaginal infections with this organism, probably acquired by fecal contamination of the vaginal atrium.

DIAGRAM 5–8. *Balantidium coli* (ciliate)

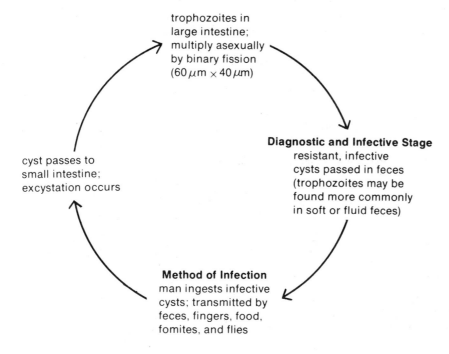

trophozoites in large intestine; multiply asexually by binary fission (60 μm × 40 μm)

Diagnostic and Infective Stage
resistant, infective cysts passed in feces (trophozoites may be found more commonly in soft or fluid feces)

Method of Infection
man ingests infective cysts; transmitted by feces, fingers, food, fomites, and flies

cyst passes to small intestine; excystation occurs

METHOD OF DIAGNOSIS

Identification of trophozoites or cysts in feces or intestinal mucosa.

DIAGNOSTIC STAGE

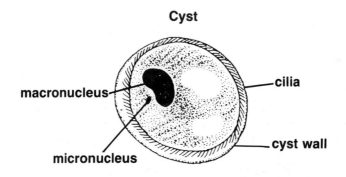

Cyst

macronucleus

cilia

micronucleus

cyst wall

40 to 50 μm

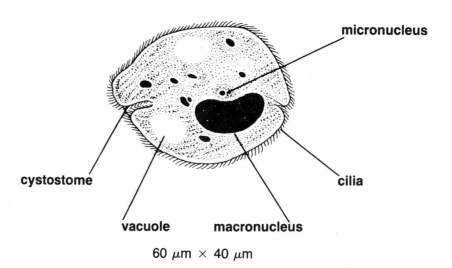

Trophozoite

micronucleus

cystostome

cilia

vacuole   macronucleus

60 μm × 40 μm

DISEASE NAMES

Balantidiasis, balantidial dysentery

MAJOR PATHOLOGY AND SYMPTOMS

May be asymptomatic. Abdominal discomfort with mild to moderate chronic recurrent diarrhea or acute dysentery. Healthy person less likely to develop illness.

TREATMENT

1. tetracycline
2. iodoquinol of metronidazole

DISTRIBUTION

Worldwide, especially in tropics where malnutrition is widespread.

Of Note

1. Pig feces are regarded as a potential source of infection.
2. *B. coli* may invade the intestinal mucosa causing hyperemia and hemorrhage of the bowel surface but does not spread via blood stream.
3. Largest protozoa and the only ciliated protozoa to infect humans.

CLASS SPOROZOA

TABLE 5–3. Sporozoans

Order	Scientific Name	Common Name
Eucoccidiida	*Plasmodium vivax* (plaz-mo'dee-um/vye'vacks)	benign tertian malaria
Eucoccidiida	*Plasmodium falciparum* (plaz-mo'dee-um/fal-sip'uh-rum)	malignant tertian malaria
Eucoccidiida	*Plasmodium malariae* (plaz-mo'dee-um/ma-lair'ee-ee)	quartan malaria
Eucoccidiida	*Plasmodium ovale* (plaz-mo'dee-um/ovay'lee)	ovale malaria
Eucoccidiida	*Toxoplasma gondii* (tock"so-plaz'muh/gon'dee-eye)	toxoplasma
Eucoccidiida	*Sarcocystis* spp. (sahr"ko-sis-tis)	none
Eucoccidiida	*Isospora belli* (eye"sos'puh-ruh/bell-eye)	none
Eucoccidiida	*Cryptosporidium* spp. (krip"toe-spor-i'dee-um)	none
Piroplasmida	*Babesia* spp. (bab-ee"zee'-uh)	none
Uncertain	*Pneumocystis carinii* (new-moe"sis-tis/kah-reye"nee-eye)	none

Sporozoan parasites are obligate endoparasitic protozoa with no apparent organelles of locomotion. This class includes some of the most important and widespread parasites of humans, including those that cause malaria and toxoplasmosis (see Table 5–3). Most species produce a spore form that is infective for the definitive host after it is ingested or after injection by a biting arthropod vector. All genera have a life cycle that includes both sexual (**gametocyte** production and **sporogony**) and asexual (**schizogony**) phases of reproduction. Most have a two-host life cycle.

The genus *Plasmodium* includes the sporozoa that causes human malaria. The asexual cycle (schizogony) begins when the infected female *Anopheles* mosquito (the definitive host) bites a human and injects infective **sporozoites,** which then enter cutaneous blood vessels. The sporozoites travel via blood and invade liver cells. Each becomes a **cryptozoite,** reproducing by asexual division and forming many **merozoites.** This is the exoerythrocytic cycle and is completed in 1 to 2 weeks.

The merozoites escape from the liver cells and invade circulating red blood cells (RBC). Merozoites entering RBCs become trophozoites (also known as ring forms) which then mature through the **schizont** stage in 36 to 72 hours. Each schizont produces 6 to 24 new merozoites. The timing and number of new merozoites produced depend on the species of *Plasmodium*. When the schizont is mature, the RBC ruptures, releasing the merozoites, which in turn invade new RBCs. This cycle of RBC invasion, schizogony, and cell rupture repeats over and over again. This is the erythrocytic cycle: merozoite enters RBC→trophozoite→schizont→RBC rupture→merozoite release. Each cycle induces a **paroxysm** as toxic materials are released from the many ruptured RBCs. The paroxysm begins suddenly and is characterized by a 10- to 15-minute (or longer) period of shaking chills followed by a feverish period lasting from 2 to 6 hours or more. The patient begins sweating profusely as the temperature returns to normal. The paroxysm is, in part, an allergic response to released parasitic antigens.

Later in the infection some merozoites develop into microgametocytes (male sex cells) and macrogametocytes (female sex cells). The sexual cycle (sporogony) begins when gametocytes are ingested by an *Anopheles* mosquito (definitive host) as she takes a blood meal from an infected person. The **gametes** unite in the stomach of the mosquito, forming a motile **zygote** (the **öokinete**), which then moves through and encysts on the mosquito's stomach wall. After further maturation to an **öocyst,** infective sporozoites are released from the öocyst; these migrate to the mosquito's salivary glands. The mosquito bite will now be infective to the next human victim. Infective sporozoites will enter via the saliva of the mosquito and travel to the liver, and the cycle begins again. Malaria can also be transmitted via blood transfusion and from contaminated needles used by drug addicts.

Drug-resistant strains of *Plasmodium* spp. and insecticide-resistant strains of mosquitoes, which have recently and rapidly evolved, pose major problems in controlling the disease worldwide. Control measures have essentially eliminated the disease from some countries, including the United States, but it is still a major problem in Africa, Asia, Central and South Americas, and areas of Europe and could potentially be reintroduced into controlled areas.

Of the four species included in the life cycle diagram, *P. falciparum* is the most deadly. These parasites promote physiological changes of the red cell (which develop a "knobby" surface) causing agglutination and lysis. Furthermore, schizogony takes place in the capillaries and blood sinuses of the brain, visceral organs, and placenta, with infected cells tending to adhere to one another and to the surrounding vessel walls. Vessels become plugged, causing local damage to the organ. Symptoms vary according to the degree of tissue anoxia and rupture of blocked capillaries. Many uninfected red cells also lyse during a paroxysm. Normal host responses to cell remnants and other parasitic debris lead to more lysis and enlargement of the spleen and liver. Other complications include renal failure caused by renal anoxia. The sudden massive intravascular lysis of RBCs followed by hemoglobin passage in urine (black water fever) is related to treatment with quinine in susceptible individuals. The most severe complication, cerebral malaria, occurs when vessels in the brain become affected. Coma and death may follow.

Pathology caused by the other *Plasmodium* spp. is less severe, primarily because these parasites are not able to invade red cells of all ages, as are *P. falciparum* parasites. Additionally, they do not cause changes to the red cell membrane as seen with *P. falciparum*. Merozoites of *P. malaria* can invade only older cells, but those of *P. vivax* and *P. ovale* infect reticulocytes. Inasmuch as these cell populations are small at any given time, the infection is limited by the environment provided by the host. *P. falciparum* can infect cells of all ages.

P. vivax is the most widely disseminated and most prevalent of the malarias. There is repeated exoerythrocytic development in the liver so that *P. vivax* can cause relapses with erythrocytic cycles starting again years after the initial infection sequence. This is thought to be due to **hypnozoites** in the liver.

DIAGRAM 5–9. *Plasmodium* species (malaria)

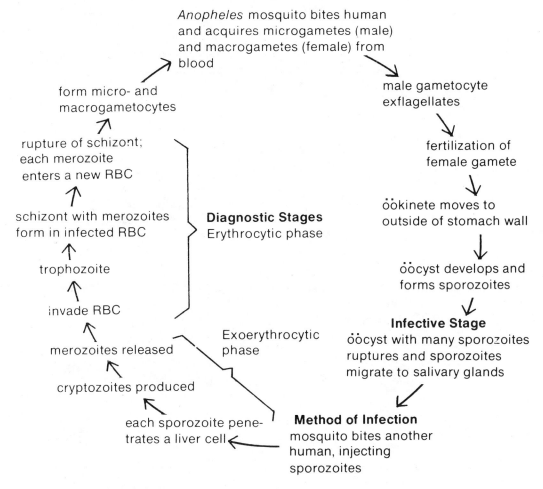

Anopheles mosquito bites human and acquires microgametes (male) and macrogametes (female) from blood

form micro- and macrogametocytes

rupture of schizont; each merozoite enters a new RBC

schizont with merozoites form in infected RBC

trophozoite

invade RBC

Diagnostic Stages
Erythrocytic phase

merozoites released

cryptozoites produced

each sporozoite penetrates a liver cell

Exoerythrocytic phase

male gametocyte exflagellates

fertilization of female gamete

öökinete moves to outside of stomach wall

öocyst develops and forms sporozoites

Infective Stage
öocyst with many sporozoites ruptures and sporozoites migrate to salivary glands

Method of Infection
mosquito bites another human, injecting sporozoites

METHOD OF DIAGNOSIS

Demonstration and identification of trophozoites, schizonts, or gametocytes in peripheral blood. Ideally, blood should be drawn between paroxysms as the greatest number of parasites is likely to be present in the specimen at this time. The cycle of paroxysms is given below. Negative morning and afternoon thick-stained smears for three consecutive days during symptoms indicate no infection. Serology is helpful.

DIAGNOSTIC STAGES

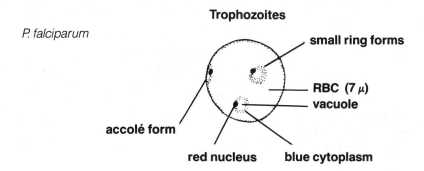

P. falciparum

Trophozoites

small ring forms

RBC (7 μ)

vacuole

accolé form

red nucleus   blue cytoplasm

**Gametocyte
(crescent-shaped)**

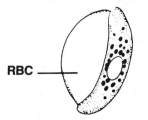

RBC ——

Note: Advanced trophozoites
and schizonts
generally not seen in
peripheral blood

P. malariae

**Trophozoite
(single ring)**

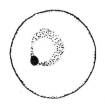

Note: Trophozoite
forms band across RBC
during early schizogony.

**Schizont
(6–12 merozoites)**

**Gametocyte
(ovoid)**

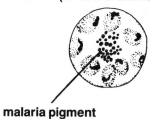

—— RBC

malaria pigment

P. vivax

**Trophozoite
(single ring)**

Reticulocyte
(immature RBC 7–10 μ) ——

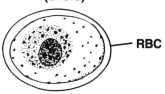

Schüffner's dots

Note: Single ring,
one third diameter of
an RBC; invades only
immature RBCs so that
large bluish cells are
parasitized.
RBC shows red-stained
Schüffner's dots which
become visible between
15 and 20 hours following
invasion of the cell.

**Schizont
(12–24 merozoites)**

Note: Trophozoite is very
ameboid and assumes bizarre
shapes during early schizogony.

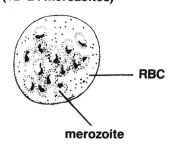

—— RBC

merozoite

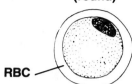

**Gametocyte
(round)**

RBC

P. ovale **(rare)**	**Note: Single ring, one third diameter of RBC. RBC is oval, shows Schüffner's dots.**

DISEASE NAMES

		Cyclic Paroxysms
P. falciparum	malignant malaria	every 36 to 48 hours
P. vivax	tertian malaria	every 48 hours
P. malariae	quartan malaria	every 72 hours
P. ovale	ovale malaria	every 48 hours

MAJOR PATHOLOGY AND SYMPTOMS

All cause splenic enlargement, fever and chills paroxysms, pains in the joints, and anemia from red cell destruction. Malaria pigment is deposited in tissues. *P. falciparum* infection can cause high fever, bloody urine, massive hemolysis, and brain damage from clumping of RBCs and resultant blocking of capillaries; subsequent rapid death can occur. High IgM and IgG levels suggest current or recurrent infections; elevated IgG alone indicates past infection. Quartan malaria nephropathy is immunopathologic from immune complex deposition in kidneys. *P. falciparum* infections result in massive hemolysis, hemoglobinuria (black water fever), and renal failure. Suspicion and response must be high for the diagnosis of malaria when patient who has visited or lived in malarious area shows compatible illness, because death can occur quickly if treatment is delayed.

TREATMENT

Chloroquin, quinine, pyrimethamine, sulfadiazine, tetracycline

DISTRIBUTION

P. falciparum and *P. malariae*—tropics
P. vivax—tropics, subtropics, and some temperate regions; most common species
P. ovale—West Africa
P. vivax and *P. falciparum* account for over 95 percent of infections; primarily a rural disease; incidence seriously increasing

OF NOTE

1. *P. vivax* and *P. ovale* may cause relapses years later because of secondary exo-erythrocytic cycles (hypnozoites in liver); primaquine is used to kill the liver phase organisms of malaria.
2. *P. vivax* invades reticulocytes preferentially; therefore, counterstaining blood for reticulocytes can aid identification.
3. Inherited glucose-6 phosphate dehydrogenase deficiency and hemoglobin gene alterations (such as sickle cell inheritance) may play an evolutionary role in survival of humans in endemic areas, inasmuch as these genetic variants are incompatible with parasite survival.
4. Presence of *P. falciparum* schizonts in peripheral blood indicates very grave prognosis.
5. *P. malariae* may also cause a relapse years later.

SUBCLASS COCCIDIA

DIAGRAM 5–10. Life Cycle of Coccidian Parasites

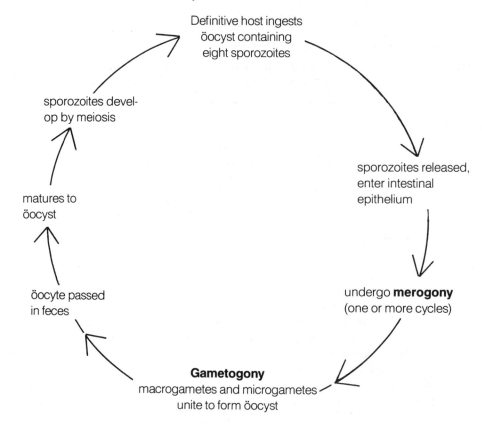

The next three genera of sporozoans discussed belong to the subclass **Coccidia;** schizogony occurs in a variety of nucleated cells of many species of mammal and birds, and sporogony occurs in the intestinal mucosa of the definitive host. Infective öocysts are passed in feces.

Toxoplasma gondii is a sporozoan parasite that infects and undergoes schizogony in all nucleated cells of almost all animals and birds. The domestic cat, however, has been cited as the definitive host for this parasite, and in the cat, it is an intestinal parasite, with both schizogony and sporogony occurring in the intestinal mucosa (the enteric cycle). Öocysts are shed in cat feces, and these become infective within several days for a variety of vertebrate intermediate hosts. Humans become infected by ingesting the infective öocyst in food or drink or by accidental means (e.g., from contaminated soil or cat litter). Initially, *Toxoplasma* divides mitotically in the tissues of humans as **tachyzoites,** which assume a crescentlike appearance in tissue fluids. It can also form **pseudocysts** (groups of **bradyzoites**) in brain and other tissues where viable toxoplasmas may remain for long periods of time, being held in check by the host's immune system.

The infection in humans is usually asymptomatic; however, it may be highly symptomatic in early infections and can mimic a variety of other infections such as infectious mononucleosis. A serious concern is that *Toxoplasma* may be transmitted across the placenta to a fetus in a mother who acquires her first infection during pregnancy. It can cause death of the fetus, mental retardation, or blindness later in life. Other sources of infection for humans in addition to ingestion of öocysts from cat feces or from transplacental infection are ingestion of undercooked meat containing calcified pseudocysts or milk containing trachyzoites. The cat becomes infected by eating infective öocysts (which are viable for up to a year in moist soil) or tissues of infected small animals. Hand-mouth transfer of öocysts from infected soil can cause infection in humans.

Diagnosis is made clinically by evaluating symptoms such as enlarged lymph nodes, by mouse inoculation with tissue such as lymph node or tonsil, by serology such as the Sabin-Feldman dye test, or by newer and recommended indirect fluorescent antibody or other specific serology techniques. With serology procedures, look for rising titres over time.

TREATMENT

1. pyrimethamine and sulfadiazine (add folinic acid in an immunosupressed host)
2. spiramycin

Several species of *Sarcocystis* have a similar life cycle to *Toxoplasma* in which pseudocysts are found in human or animal muscle tissue. These cause little pathology. The definitive host for *Sarcocystis* is the dog or cat that sheds infective öocysts in feces.

There is one pathogenic coccidian for which the human is the definitive host in which both schizogony and sporogony accompanied by mild pathology occur in the gastrointestinal tract of the infected human. This species is *Isospora belli*. Characteristic öocysts can be found in infected human feces. The öocysts of *I. belli* in a fresh fecal specimen are transparent, measuring 30 μm $\times$ 12μm, and are immature (containing a single mass of protoplasm called the sporoblast) or, rarely, developing (containing two sporoblasts). Within 18 to 36 hours after feces are passed, each of the two sporoblasts develops a cyst wall and contains four sausage-shaped infective sporozoites. Full maturation takes 4 to 5 days.

This parasite is found worldwide, and transmission to humans is direct via sporulated öocysts in fecally contaminated food or water. Cattle and pigs serve as intermediate hosts. Human infection can cause anorexia, nausea, abdominal pain and diarrhea, and possible malabsorption. Öocysts are readily recoverable with the zinc sulfate flotation technique and stain well with iodine.

TREATMENT

Trimethoprim and sulfamethoxazole

For the sporozoans of the *Babesia species* (sublcass *Piroplasmia*), ticks are the definitive hosts, and occasional tick-borne human infections have been reported. In humans, the organisms multiply in red blood cells and are generally pear-shaped (2 to 4 μm). They usually lie in pairs at an acute angle or as a tetrad in a cross formation. In examining stained thick and thin blood smears, care must be taken not to confuse these with malaria ring forms of *Plasmodium falciparum*. Clinical signs follow the bite of an infected tick in about 2 to 3 weeks and resemble symptoms of malaria, with a possible accompanying hemolytic anemia and mild spleen and liver disease.

Pneumocystis carinii is the causative agent of atypical interstitial plasma-cell pneumonia (PCP). The classification of this parasite and its life cycle is uncertain. This organism is endemic in many parts of the world and can produce pneumonia, particularly in infants and in patients with immunologic disorders such as AIDS or those receiving immunosuppressive therapy.

The organism may be demonstrated in several morphologic forms intracellulary and extracellularly in lung biopsies or in aspirates stained with silver methenamine. The thick-walled cyst form (7 to 10 μm) contains four to eight intracystic bodies (sporozoites). The organism may appear as a single pleomorphic form (2 to 5 μm) with a double outer membrane. Lung tissue assumes a honeycomb appearance. Direct contact transmission between humans by pulmonary droplets is probable. Clinical cases of pneumocystis pneumonia generally occur only in those with a predisposing debilitated state. Prognosis is poor.

TREATMENT

Trimethroprim and sulfamethoxazole or pentamidine isothionate

The genus *Cryptosporidium* is a coccidian protozoan. This parasite invades the gastro-intestinal mucosal surface of many vertebrate hosts including humans. Both trophozoites and schizonts are attached to the host-cell membrane. Eight merozoites develop within the schizont and on maturation, are released to begin a new schizonic cycle or to initiate a sexual cycle. Macro- and microgametocytes become mature gametes. Sexual union forms an oocyte which then developes into an öocyst. The entire life cycle occurs within a single host. Infection is probably acquired from food or water contaminated with öocysts in feces from an animal reservoir host.

Human infection, first reported in 1976, is infrequent and occurs primarily in patients who have compromised immune systems. The symptom found in all reported cases is acute diarrhea. The disease is self-limiting in patients with normal immune systems and lasts from 1 to 2 weeks. Immunodeficient patients, such as those with AIDS and those receiving immunosuppressant drugs, may have chronic diarrhea.

The organism is identified by electron microscopy and by Giemsa-stained smears of biopsy material from the jejunum. Stained cells containing *Cryptosporidium* spp. appear as spherical bodies measuring 2 to 4 μm in diameter. Trophozoites, schizonts, microgemetocytes and macrogametocytes can be distinguished when using the electron microscope.

TREATMENT

Spiromycin (experimental)

Isospora belli

Mature Öocyst

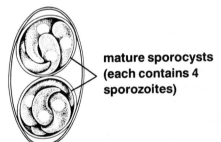

mature sporocysts
(each contains 4
sporozoites)

30 × 15 μm

Babesia microti

Trophozoites

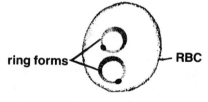

ring forms — RBC

2–5 μm

Pneumocystis carinii

Mature Cyst

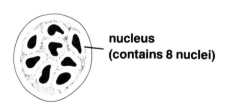

nucleus
(contains 8 nuclei)

7 to 10 μm

Table 5—4 reviews the life cycles and other important information about the protozoa. Study these carefully before taking the chapter post-test.

TABLE 5—4. Pathogenic Protozoa

Scientific and Common Name	Epidemiology	Disease Producing Form and Its Location in Hosts	How Infection Occurs	Major Disease Manifestations, Diagnostic Stage, and Specimen of Choice
Entamoeba histolytica (amebic dysentery)	World-wide	Trophozoites in large intestinal mucosa, liver, or other tissues	Ingestion of cyst in fecally contaminated food or water	Enteritis with abdominal pain and bloody dysentery Diagnosis: cysts and trophozoites in feces
Acanthamoeba spp. (chronic meningoencephalitis)	World-wide	Trophozoites and cysts in tissues of brain, eye, skin, etc.	Accidental entrance through skin lesion	Slow disease development (over 10 days)
Naegleria fowleri (primary amoebic meningoencephalitis)	World-wide	Amoebic trophozoites in brain	Accidental entrance of free-living water-borne trophozoites through nasopharynx mucosa	Rapid death
Dientamoeba fragilis (none)	World-wide	Trophozoites in large intestine	Ingestion of trophozoite (?)	Diarrhea Diagnosis: trophozoites in feces (no cysts formed)
Giardia lamblia (traveler's diarrhea)	World-wide	Trophozoites in large intestinal mucosa	Ingestion of cysts in fecally contaminated food or water	Mild to severe dysentery; malabsorption syndrome Diagnosis: cysts and trophozoites in feces
Trichomonas vaginalis (trich)	World-wide	Trophozoites in urethra or vagina	Sexual contact	Irritating, frothy vaginal discharge; men usually asymptomatic

TABLE 5–4. *Continued*

Scientific and Common Name	Epidemiology	Disease Producing Form and Its Location in Host	How Infection Occurs	Major Disease Manifestations, Diagnostic Stage, and Specimen of Choice
Trichomonas vaginalis (trich). *continued*				Diagnosis: trophozoites in urine or vaginal smear (no cysts formed)
Leishmania tropica (oriental sore)	Mediterranean area, Asia, Africa, Central America	Amastigotes in macrophages of skin lesion	Bite of *Phlebotomus* spp. (sandfly)	Self-healing skin lesion Diagnosis: amastigotes in macrophages around lesion
Leishmania mexicana (New World cutaneous leishmaniasis)	Mexico, Central and South America	Amastigotes in macrophages of skin lesions	Bite of *Phlebotomus* spp.	Self-healing skin lesion; some species cause diffuse cutaneous leishmaniasis
Leishmania braziliensis (New World leishmaniasis; espundia)	Central and South America especially Brazil	Amastigotes in macrophages of skin lesion and mucocutaneous tissue	Bite of *Phlebotomus* spp.	Self-healing skin lesion, later ulceration of cephalic mucocutaneous tissue Diagnosis: recovery of amastigotes from lesion
Leishmania donovani (kala-azar)	Mediterranean area, Asia, Africa, South America	Amastigotes in macrophages in skin lesion and somatic organs	Bite of *Phlebotomus* spp.	Initial skin lesion, later daily double-spiking fever, enlarged liver and spleen, death in late stages Diagnosis: L.D. bodies in early lesion, organ tissue biopsy later

TABLE 5–4. *Continued*

Scientific and Common Name	Epidemio-logy	Disease Producing Form and Its Location in Host	How Infection Occurs	Major Disease Manifestations, Diagnostic Stage, and Specimen of Choice
Trypanosoma gambiense (sleeping sickness)	West Africa	Trypomastigote in blood, lymph nodes, later in CNS	Bite of Glossina spp. (tsetse fly)	Fever, lymphadenopathy (Winterbottom's sign), enlarged spleen and liver, lethargy and death Diagnosis: trypomastigotes in blood smear, CSF
Trypanosoma rhodesiense (sleeping sickness)	East Africa	Trypomastigote in blood lymph nodes, later in CNS	Bite of *Glossina* spp. (tsetse fly)	Fever, lymphadenopathy (Winterbottom's sign), enlarged spleen and liver, lethargy and death Course more acute and fatal than *T. gambiense* Diagnosis: trypomastigotes in blood smear
Trypanosoma cruzi (Chagas' disease)	South America	C-shaped trypomastigote and epimastigote forms early in blood; later L.D. bodies in heart and other tissues	Infected feces of *Triatoma* spp. (kissing bug) rubbed into bite site	Fever, enlarged spleen and liver, Romaña's sign (edema around eyes), chronic damage to heart and alimentary tract Acute death, especially in children Diagnosis: trypomastigotes in blood; xenodiagnosis
Balantidium coli (balantidial dysentery)	Worldwide	Trophozoites in large intestinal mucosa	Ingestion of cysts in fecally	Moderate or mild dysentery

TABLE 5–4. *Continued*

Scientific and Common Name	Epidemiology	Disease Producing Form and Its Location in Host	How Infection Occurs	Major Disease Manifestations, Diagnostic Stage, and Specimen of Choice
			contaminated food or water	Diagnosis: trophozoites or cysts in feces
Plasmodium vivax (benign tertian malaria)	Tropics, subtropics, some temperate regions	Schizogony and gametocytes in RBCs	*Anopheles* spp. mosquito transmits sporozoites	Cyclic fever, chills, enlarged spleen, parasites in red blood cells Diagnosis: malarial forms in blood smear
Plasmodium malariae (quartan malaria)	Tropics	Schizogony and gametocytes in RBCs	*Anopheles* spp. mosquito transmits sporozoites	Cyclic fever, chills, enlarged spleen, parasites in RBCs; relapses Diagnosis: malarial forms in blood smear
Plasmodium falciparum (malignant malaria)	Tropics	Trophozoites and gametocytes in peripheral RBCs	*Anopheles* spp. mosquito transmits sporozoites	Cyclic fever, chills, enlarged spleen, parasites in RBCs Blackwater fever from hemoglobin in urine, blockage of capillaries, death Diagnosis: malarial forms in blood smear
Plasmodium ovale (ovale malaria)	West Africa	Schizogony and gametocytes in RBCs	*Anopheles* spp. mosquito transmits sporozoites	Cyclic fever, chills, enlarged spleen, parasites in RBCs Diagnosis: malarial forms in blood smear
Toxoplasma gondii (toxoplasmosis)	Worldwide	Trophozoites intracellularly in all organs;	Ingestion of oocysts; ingestion of	Fever, enlarged lymph nodes

TABLE 5–4. *Continued*

Scientific and Common Name	Epidemiology	Disease Producing Form and Its Location in Host	How Infection Occurs	Major Disease Manifestations, Diagnostic Stage, and Specimen of Choice
Toxoplasma gondii (toxoplasmosis). *continued*		pseudocysts in brain and other tissue	trophozoites or pseudocysts in undercooked meat; congenital passage of trophozoites	In fetus or neonate: damage or death Can cause acute infection in immunosuppressed patient Diagnosis: serology
Isospora belli (none)	Worldwide	Schizogony and gametogony stages in intestinal epithelium	Ingestion of infective öocysts	Diarrhea Diagnosis: oocyst and sporocysts in feces
Sarcocystis spp. (none) (zoonosis)	Worldwide	Sarcocyst in muscle	Unknown: may be by ingestion of sarcocyst from undercooked meat or öocyst	Sarcocysts (Miescher's tubes) in muscle do not generally cause problems Diagnosis: tissue biopsy
Pneumocystis carinii (none)	Europe, Asia, U.S.A.	Cysts in lungs	Unknown	Interstitial plasma cell pneumonia, in immunosuppressed patients. Frequently seen in AIDS patients. Diagnosis: cysts or pleomorphic forms in bronchioalveolar lavage or transbronchial biopsy. Honeycomb appearance of lung tissue.

TABLE 5–4. *Continued*

Scientific and Common Name	Epidemio-logy	Disease Producing Form and Its Location in Host	How Infec-tion Occurs	Major Disease Manifestations, Diagnostic Stage, and Specimen of Choice
Cryptospori-dium spp. (none)	Worldwide	Invades GI tract mucosa	Unknown; may be by ingestion of fecally contaminated food or water	Diarrhea Diagnosis: tropho-zoites and schiz-onts in biopsy of jejunum
Babesia spp. (none) (zoonosis)	Worldwide	*Babesia* tropho-zoites in RBC	tick bite	Fever; symptoms can resemble malaria Diagnosis: tropho-zoites in blood smear

Consult Color Plates 72 to 126.

You have now completed the section on *Protozoa*. After reviewing this material with the aid of your learning objectives, proceed to the post-test.

BIBLIOGRAPHY

INTESTINAL PROTOZOA

AREAN, VM AND KOPPISCH, E: *Balantidiosis: A review and report cases.* Am J Pathol 32:1089, 1956.

BABB, RR, PECK, OC, AND VESCIA, FG: *Giardiasis: A cause of traveler's diarrhea.* JAMA 217:1359, 1971.

BRANDBORG, LL, GOLDBERG, SB, AND BRIEDENBOCH, WC: *Human coccidiosis—A possi-ble cause of malabsorption. The life cycle in small bowel mucosal biopsies as a di-agnostic feature.* N Engl J Med 283:1306, 1970.

ELSDON-DEW, R: *The epidemiology of amoebiasis.* In DAWES, B (ED): *Advances in Parasi-tology,* Vol 6. Academic Press, New York, 1968, pp 1–62.

ELSDON-DEW, R: *Parasitic infections and the genitourinary tract.* Practitioner 214:75, 1975.

HOSKINS, LC, WINAWER, SJ, BROITMAN, SA, ET AL: *Clinical giardiasis and intestinal mal-absorption.* Gastroenterology 53:265, 1967.

KNIGHT, R AND WRIGHT, SC: *Progress report: Intestinal protozoa.* Gut 19:940, 1978.

KROGSTAD, DJ, SPENCER, HC, AND HEALY, GR: *Current concepts in parasitology: Amebi-asis.* N Engl J Med 298:262, 1978.

MAHMOUD, AAF AND WARREN, KS: *Algorithms in the diagnosis and management of exotic diseases. II. Giardiasis.* J Infect Dis 131:621,1975.

PRITCHARD, JH, WINSTON, MA, BERGER, HG, ET AL: *Diagnosis of focal hepatic lesions. Combined radioisotope and ultrasound techniques.* JAMA 229:1463, 1974.

SCHULTZ, MG: *Giardiasis.* JAMA 233:1383, 1975.

Atrial and Blood Protozoa

Atias, A, Neghme, A, Aquirre MacKay, L, and Jarpa, S: *Mega-esophagus, megacolon and Chagas' disease in Chile.* Gastroenterology 44:433, 1963.

Brown, MT: *Trichomoniasis.* Practitioner 207:639, 1972.

Cohen, S: *Immunity to malaria.* Proc Roy Soc Lond (Biol) 203:323, 1979.

Convit, J, Pinardi, ME, and Rondon, AJ: *Diffuse cutaneous leishmaniasis: A disease due to an immunologic defect of the host.* Trans Roy Soc Trop Med Hyg 66:603, 1972.

Cossio, PM, Diez, C, Szarfman, A, et al: *Chagasic cardiopathy. Demonstration of a serum gamma globulin factor which reacts with endocardium and vascular structures.* Circulation 49:13, 1974.

Garnham, PCC: *Malaria Parasites and Other Haemosporidia.* Blackwell Scientific Publications, Oxford, 1966.

Goodwin, LG: *The pathology of African trypanosomiasis.* Trans Roy Soc Trop Med Hyg 65:797, 1970.

Grunwaldt, E: *Babesiosis on Shelter Island.* NY State J Med 77:1320, 1977.

Hubsch, RM, Sulzer, AJ, and Kagan, IG: *Evaluation of an autoimmune type antibody in the sera of patients with Chagas' disease.* J Parasitol 62:523, 1976.

Lumsden, WHR and Evans, DA: *Biology of the Kinetoplastida.* Vol 1. Academic Press, New York, 1976.

Luzzatto, L, Usanga, EA, and Reddy, S: *Glucose-6 phosphate dehydrogenase deficient red cells: Resistance to infection with malarial parasites.* Science 164:839, 1969.

Mahmoud, AAF and Warren, KS: *Algorithms in the diagnosis and management of exotic diseases, IV. American trypanosomiasis.* J Infect Dis 132:121, 1975.

Marsden, PD: *Current concepts in parasitology: Leishmaniasis.* N Engl J Med 300:350, 1979.

Miller, LH, Mason, SJ, Dvorak, JA, et al: *Erythrocyte receptors for (Plasmodium knowlesi) malaria: Duffy blood group determinants.* Science 189:561, 1975.

Pan American Health Organization: *Malaria: Growing alert.* (Editorial) Bull Pen Am Health Org 12:271, 1978.

Szarfman, A, Khoury, EL, Cossio, PM, et al: *Investigation of the EVI antibody in parasitic diseases other than American trypanosomiasis. An anti-skeletal muscle antibody in leishmaniasis.* Am J Trop Med Hyg 24:19, 1975.

Other Protozoa

Babb, RR, Differding, JT, and Trollope, ML: *Cryptosporidia enteritis in a health professional athlete.* Am J Gastroenterol 77:833–834.

Broadduc, C, et al: *Bronchoalveolar lavage and transbronchial biopsy for the diagnosis of pulmonary infections in the acquired immunodeficiency syndrome.* Ann Intern Med 102:747–752, 1985.

Bryan, RT and Wilson, M: *Clinical Casebook: Toxoplasmosis.* Laboratory Management 26(8):40, 1988.

Bunyarartvej, S, Bunyawongwiroj, P, and Nitiyanant, P: *Human intestinal sarcosporidiosis: Report of six cases.* Am J Trop Med Hyg 31:36–41, 1982.

Camargo, ME, et al: *Immunoglobulin G and immunoglobulin M enzyme-linked immunosorbent assays and defined toxoplasmosis serological patterns.* Infect Immunol 21:55, 1978.

Carter, RF: *Primary amoebic meningoencephalitis. An appraisal of present knowledge.* Trans Roy Soc Trop Med Hyg 66:193, 1972.

Centers for Disease Control: *Primary amebic meningoencephalitis: California, Florida, New York.* MMWR 27:343, 1978.

Cursons, RT, Brown, TJ, and Keyes, EA: *Virulence of pathogenic free-living amebae.* J Parasitol 64:744, 1978.

Frenkel, JL: *Toxoplasmosis and pneumocystosis: Clinical and laboratory aspects in im-*

munocompetent and compromised hosts. In PRIER, JE AND FRIEDMAN, H (EDS): *Opportunistic Pathogens.* University Park Press, Baltimore, 1974, pp 203–259.

GREAVES, T AND STRIGLE, S: *The recognition of Pneumocystis carinii in routine Papanicolaou stained smears.* Acta Cytol 29:714–720, 1985.

KIM, HK AND HUGHES, WT: *Comparison of methods for the identification of Pneumocystis carinii in pulmonary aspirates.* Am J Clin Pathol 60:462, 1973.

MARKUS, MB: *Sarcocystis and sarcocystosis in domestic animals and man.* Adv Vet Sci Comp Med 22:159, 1978.

MURRAY, J, ET AL: *Pulmonary complications of the acquired immunodeficiency syndrome: Report of a National Heart, Lung and Blood Institute Workshop.* N Engl J Med 310:1682–1688, 1984.

NATIONAL CANCER INSTITUTE: *Monograph No. 43. Symposium on Pneumocystis Carinii Infection.* U.S. Dept. H.E.W., P.H.S., I.I.H., 1976.

PITCHENIK, A, ET AL: *Sputum examination for the diagnosis of Pneumocystis carinii pneumoniia in the acquired immunodeficiency syndrome.* Am Rev Respir Dis 133:226–229, 1986.

ZOONOSES

COATNEY, GR: *The simian malarias: Zoonosis, anthroponosis or both?* Am J Trop Med Hyg 20:795, 1971.

LEVINE, ND: *Protozoan parasites of nonhuman primates as zoonotic agents.* Lab Animal Care 20:371, 1970.

POST-TEST

1. Matching: select the one best answer: (**36 points**)

   a. _____ malaria parasite with 6–12 mero-zoites in the schizont
   b. _____ C- or U-shaped body with a large kinetoplast
   c. _____ large kidney-shaped nucleus
   d. _____ trophozoite ingests red blood cells
   e. _____ large glycogen vacuole
   f. _____ schizonts not seen in peripheral blood
   g. _____ pseudocysts in brain
   h. _____ nonpathogenic
   i. _____ öocysts found in human feces
   j. _____ commonly causes relapses of malaria
   k. _____ transmitted by tsetse fly
   l. _____ pathogenic intestinal flagellate

   1. *Isospora belli*
   2. *Toxoplasma gondii*
   3. *Plasmodium vivax*
   4. *Plasmodium malariae*
   5. *Plasmodium falciparum*
   6. *Trypanosoma gambiense*
   7. *Trypanosoma cruzi*
   8. *Entamoeba histolytica*
   9. *Entamoeba hartmanni*
   10. *Endolimax nana*
   11. *Iodamoeba bütschlii*
   12. *Giardia lamblia*
   13. *Trichomonas vaginalis*
   14. *Balantidium coli*

2. How would you differentiate *Entamoeba histolytica* from *Endamoeba coli* in a fecal smear? (**9 points**)

3. Define: (**20 points**)

   a. trophozoite
   b. cyst
   c. sporozoite
   d. schizogony
   e. carrier

   f. öocyst
   g. pseudocyst
   h. L.D. body
   i. paroxysm
   j. atrium

4. State method of infection for each of the following diseases: (**20 points**)

   a. Kala azar
   b. Giardiasis
   c. Chagas' disease
   d. toxoplasmosis
   e. trichomonal urethritis

   f. balantidial dysentery
   g. babesiosis
   h. malaria
   i. sleeping sickness
   j. cutaneous leishmaniasis

5. Draw the ring form in a red blood cell for each of the following: (**15 points**)

   a. *Plasmodium vivax*   b. *Plasmodium malariae*   c. *Plasmodium falciparum*

ARTHROPODA

LEARNING OBJECTIVES

Upon completion of this chapter, the student will be able to

1. state the criteria used for taxonomic classification of the Arthropoda.
2. state the general description of each order of Arthropoda that contain genera of medical importance.
3. state the definitions of terminology specific for Arthropoda.
4. state the definitions of complete and incomplete metamorphosis and give examples of each.
5. identify Arthropoda to class by morphologic criteria.
6. differentiate between the Acarina and Insecta.
7. describe the type of life cycle for each Arthropoda class.
8. contrast the role of Arthropoda as intermediate hosts rather than as transport hosts for various parasites and microorganisms.
9. identify the specific genus of Arthropoda serving as the required intermediate host for various helminth and protozoal infections.
10. given an illustration or photograph (or actual specimen with sufficient laboratory experience), identify diagnostic stages of Arthropoda.
11. discuss the problems caused by the Arthropoda that have an impact on humans, and propose solutions for these problems.
12. propose method(s) of prevention of infestations caused by arthropods.
13. propose methods of control of Arthropoda based upon life cycles.

The phylum **Arthropoda** includes the segmented invertebrates that have a protective **chitinous exoskeleton** and bilaterally paired jointed appendages. The head has structures adapted for sensory and chewing or piercing functions. Eyes are single or compound. Digestive, respiratory, excretory, and nervous systems are present. The body cavity (the hemocele) is an open space filled with a bloodlike substance.

This large group is divided into five classes, and three of these, **Insecta, Arachnida,** and **Crustacea,** contain most of the medically important arthropods. The important disease-producing genera listed in Table 6–1 are members of various families. The Arthropoda is the largest phylum, containing over 80 percent of all animal life. It also directly causes or transmits over 80 percent of all diseases. It is of major economic importance to agriculture, with both beneficial and destructive effects.

All Arachnida and most Insecta develop from egg to adult by a process called **metamorphosis.** Incomplete (hemimetabolous) metamorphosis has three stages: (1) egg, (2) **nymph,** and (3) **imago,** the sexually mature adult. The nymph, a miniature adult, molts several times before it becomes an adult. The nymphal form after each molt is called an **instar.** Wings of flying insects increase in size with each instar. Lice, bugs, and arachnids are hemimetabolous.

Complete (holometabolous) metamorphosis has four stages: (1) egg, (2) larva, (3) pupa, and (4) imago. Insect larvae appear as segmented wormlike organisms and mature through a series of instars which finally enclose themselves inside a case, or **pupa.** After a time, the transformed imago emerges. Flies, mosquitoes, and fleas are holometabolous.

Development of most crustaceans is by incomplete metamorphosis; however, the names of the stages are different. Eggs hatch, releasing free-swimming **nauplius** larvae which molt several times to become mature adults. Some species, however, undergo complete metamorphosis; the nauplius larva develops into a **cypris** larva (a stage similar to the pupa), and the transformed larva emerges as an adult.

It is crucial that you understand the importance of the Arthropoda—both as parasites themselves and as vectors of other disease-causing microorganisms. While some insects and parasites of man (e.g., ectoparasites such as lice, mosquitoes, and ticks which feed on blood), other insects play an important role as vectors that transmit a variety of diseases. Elimination of the vector is a frequently attempted method of parasite control. Therefore, it is important to know which insect species comprise an integral part of a parasite's life cycle and also to understand the life cycle of the insect itself in order to initiate proper measures of control.

Mechanical transfer of infective organisms from feces or contaminated soil to food or utensils by the feet or mouth parts of insects coupled with inadequate protection of food and inadequate personal hygiene provides the means by which a person may contract an infection. Mechanical transfer implies that no further development or growth of the parasite occurs in the insect, even if the parasite is carried inside the insect and is released in the insect's feces or is injected into the host by the biting insect. A biological vector, on the other hand, requires that growth and development of the parasite occur inside the insect. Insects may serve as either definitive or intermediate hosts. The infective parasites that develop in the insect are either injected directly into a new host or, in a few species, are deposited on the host's skin.

Some pathogens can be passed from an adult insect to its offspring if the organism penetrates the egg(s) *in vivo.* This is known as transovarial transmission. If the pathogen is able to survive in each part of the cycle (egg→nymph→adult), it has been transmitted trans-stadially. The term *vertical transmission* used to describe these phenomena means that parasites are being passed from generation to generation within the same species. Certain diseases are maintained by tick vectors via vertical transmission.

Besides mechanical or biological disease transmission, other major problems caused by insects are annoyance, delayed or immediate hypersensitivity reactions to bites (including fatal anaphylaxis), blood loss, secondary bacterial infections in open insect bite sites, injection of toxins or venoms, loss of food crops, loss of animal productivity, and **myiasis.**

Myiasis is caused by larvae of non-blood sucking flies invading tissue. Eggs or larvae may be deposited directly on skin or are transferred to the body from contaminated soil. Although myiasis is more commonly seen in animals, man may serve as a host for several species. For example, the fly, *Cochliomyia hominivorax,* causes the disease known as primary screwworm. The fly is attached to open wounds or nasal drainage, where it deposits its eggs. Larvae hatch in 11 to 22 hours, invade the skin, and begin feeding on tissue. Symptoms depend on the site of invasion, but pain, swelling, and subcutaneous larval migration occur in most cases. Many other fly larvae cause similar problems worldwide, especially in children and livestock herders. Accidental ingestion of fly eggs or larvae may produce intestinal myiasis, resulting in various gastrointestinal symptoms.

Control of Arthropoda is difficult. Use of chemical sprays is widespread but has very serious consequences for the environment and other life forms, because synthetic chemicals are not biodegradable and remain in the food chain. In addition, many insecticide-resistant species of insects have evolved. Other arthropod control methods being tried include increasing natural predators, destroying breeding grounds, biologic control (e.g., releasing artificially sterilized males, as was attempted with screwworm flies), pheromone and other types of traps, introduction of a faster-breeding competitive species, and removal of host species on which the insect feeds.

There are basic morphologic differences between the classes and orders of arthropods that enable you to readily distinguish between ticks, mites, flies, mosquitoes, bugs, lice, and fleas. The upcoming section on insect morphology will present the major structural differences between the classes of medically important arthropods as well as some clinical and epidemiologic details. By studying Table 6–1, you can review those important genera of arthropods that transmit various infections to humans.

GLOSSARY

ARTHROPODA. A phylum of the animal kingdom composed of organisms having a hard, segmented exoskeleton and paired, jointed legs.

Arachnida. A class in the phylum *Arthropoda* containing ticks, mites, spiders, and scorpions.

capitulum. A collective term referring to the mouthparts of ticks and mites which extend forward from the body of the tick or mite.

chitin. A horny, insoluble polysaccharide which is the main compound found in shells of crabs, exoskeletons of insects, and other insect structures.

Crustacea. A class in the phylum *Arthropoda* including crabs, water fleas, lobsters, shrimp, barnacles, and wood lice.

ctenidium (pl. ctenidia). A spinelike process found on the head region of fleas. These comblike structures are useful in group classification. Genal ctenidia or combs are located just above the mouthparts. Pronotal combs are located immediately behind the head and extend posteriorly on the dorsal surface.

cypris. A larval resting stage in the life cycle of some crustaceans in which a metamorphosis occurs, comparable to a pupa.

ecdysis. The molting or shedding of an outer layer or covering and the development of a new one.

entomology. The branch of zoology dealing with the study of insects.

exoskeleton. A hard, chitinous structure on the outside of the body, providing support for internal organs.

imago. The sexually mature adult insect or arachnid.

Insecta. A class in the phylum *Arthropoda* containing many insect types whose bodies are divided into three distinct regions—head, thorax, and abdomen.

instar. Any one of the nymphal or larval stages between molts.

invertebrates. Animals having no spinal column.

metamorphosis. A change of shape or structure; a transition from one developmental stage to another. In simple or incomplete metamorphosis, nymphs resemble adults; in complete metamorphosis, larvae and pupae do not resemble adults.

myiasis. A condition caused by infestation of the body with fly larvae.

nauplius. The earliest and youngest larval form in the life cycle of crustaceans.

nymph. A developmental stage in the life cycle of certain arthropods which resembles the adult morphologically.

pediculosis. Infestation with lice, especially with *P. humanus.*

pupa (pl. pupae). The encased resting stage between the larva and imago stage (e.g., cocoon).

scutum. A chitinous shield or plate covering part (female) or all (male) of the dorsal surface of hard ticks.

temporary host. A host on which an arthropod (adult or larval form) resides temporarily in order to feed on blood or tissue.

DIAGRAM 6–1. Classification of Arthropods

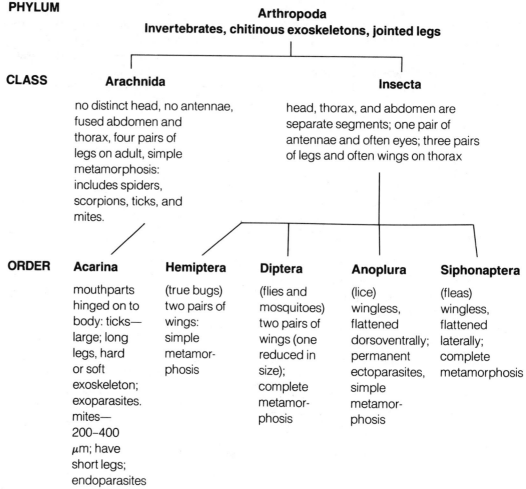

PHYLUM

Arthropoda
Invertebrates, chitinous exoskeletons, jointed legs

CLASS

Arachnida

no distinct head, no antennae, fused abdomen and thorax, four pairs of legs on adult, simple metamorphosis: includes spiders, scorpions, ticks, and mites.

Insecta

head, thorax, and abdomen are separate segments; one pair of antennae and often eyes; three pairs of legs and often wings on thorax

ORDER

Acarina

mouthparts hinged on to body: ticks— large; long legs, hard or soft exoskeleton; exoparasites. mites— 200–400 μm; have short legs; endoparasites

Hemiptera

(true bugs) two pairs of wings: simple metamorphosis

Diptera

(flies and mosquitoes) two pairs of wings (one reduced in size); complete metamorphosis

Anoplura

(lice) wingless, flattened dorsoventrally; permanent ectoparasites, simple metamorphosis

Siphonaptera

(fleas) wingless, flattened laterally; complete metamorphosis

INSECT MORPHOLOGY

CLASS INSECTA

Order Diptera (Flies and Mosquitoes)

This is the order of greatest medical importance; blood-sucking mosquitoes and flies transmit many viral, protozoan, and helminthic diseases. They are all ectoparasites as adults. One can differentiate among the dipteran insects by studying the characteristics of the parts listed and by using an indentification key in an **entomology** text or insect identification handbook.

Examine

1. antennae—number of segments, presence or absence of hairs
2. mouth parts—structures for piercing skin or sucking fluid
3. coloration and hair distribution on body
4. size and shape of body and each of the three body segments
5. morphology of eggs, larval and pupal stages
6. pattern of veins in the wings

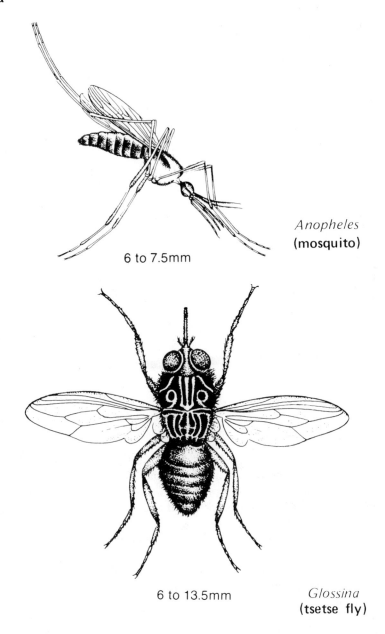

Anopheles
(mosquito)

6 to 7.5mm

6 to 13.5mm   *Glossina*
(tsetse fly)

Order Anoplura (Lice)

Lice are flattened dorsoventrally and have a three-segment body with antennae on the head and three pairs of legs extending from the middle segment (the thorax). The legs have claws on the ends for grasping body hair. Metamorphosis is simple, and the immature stages look like the adults. Lice are very host specific. The lice are permanent ectoparasites and live only on the host, surviving just briefly in the environment. Eggs (nits) are deposited on hair shafts of the host. The order Anoplura are blood-sucking lice; the mouthparts are adapted for piercing the skin and sucking blood. The head is narrower than the thorax; *Phthiris pubis* (crab louse) and *Pediculus humanus* (head and body lice) are epidemic in the United States, with at least 6 million cases annually.

Lice are transferred directly from host to host. Additionally, eggs from louse-infested clothing or other personal articles may be sources of infection. Pubic lice are usually transferred via sexual intercourse, but infections may be acquired in locker rooms from towels and from mats on gymasium floors. Symptoms of **pediculosis** include itchy papules at the site of infestation. Saliva and fecal excretions of the louse often cause a local hypersensitivity reaction which leads to inflammation. If secondary bacterial infection occurs, the lesion may resemble mange. Successful treatment requires that both eggs and motile stages are killed.

Body lice transmit *Rickettsia* spp., the causative agents of endemic typhus and trench fever. Louse-borne relapsing fever caused by *Borrelia recurrentis* is also transmitted by *pediculus humanus.*

Treatment. *Phthiris pubis:* 0.5 percent malathion lotion or 1 percent lindane. *Pediculus humanus:* (1) permethrin, (2) pyrethrin with butoxide or 0.5 percent malathion or 1 percent lindane.

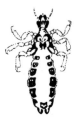

Pediculus
(body louse)

2 to 4 mm

Phthiris pubis
(crab louse)

1 mm

Order Siphonaptera (Fleas)

Fleas are flattened laterally. They, too, have three pairs of clawed legs extending from the thorax, but the rear pair are very long and adapted for jumping. The species of fleas can be differentiated by looking for the presence or absence of eyes and the genal and pronotal **ctenidia** (combs). Adult fleas suck blood and have mouth parts adapted for this purpose. Metamorphosis is complete; all stages develop to maturity in the external environment. The adult flea takes a blood meal from a temporary host and then lays eggs in dark crevices. A flea infestation must be treated by cleaning the environment as well as the host. Complete chemical control is difficult. Chemical treatment and control measures in the environment should be repeated 2 weeks later to kill larvae and adults that developed from resistant eggs.

Adult fleas may live as long as a year, and eggs may remain viable for even longer periods. The rat flea, *xenopsylla cheopis,* is known to transmit *Rickettsia typhi,* the bacteria responsible for murine typhus. The rat flea is the primary vector for the causative agent of bubonic plague, *Yersinia pestis.* Inasmuch as rats often live in colonies, fleas feed freely on various hosts. The disease is spread from rat to rat via fecal excretions deposited near flea bite sites. Plague bacilli gain entrance through the bite wound. Infected fleas crushed on the host's body also allow the bacteria to gain entrance into the rat. Bubonic plague can be found in squirrels and other small mammals as well. Control of the disease rests mainly on controlling rats and squirrels. Human cases numbered 105 in 8 western states during the 1970s. This is the largest number of cases reported in the United States of America in any decade since 1900 to 1909. Under suitable conditions this bacteria may remain infective for 5 years in dried flea feces. These facts illustrate the difficulty of controlling fleas and the diseases they transmit.

As ectoparasites, fleas cause itchy bites when they feed. Adults will usually feed several times in the same day and may move from host to host when several hosts are available. Furthermore, fleas are not very host specific. Dog and cat fleas will readily take a blood meal from humans. Although dog and cat fleas are not good transmitters of the plague bacillus, they can transmit tapeworms (*H. nana* and *H. diminuta*) to humans. The primary problem caused by these fleas is irritation with possible allergic reactions to the bites. Secondary bacterial invasion may also occur as itchy bites are scratched.

Ctenocephalides
(flea)

1.5 to 4 mm

CLASS ARACHNIDA

Order Acarina (Ticks and Mites)

The mouth parts of ticks and mites are adapted for piercing and are attached directly on the fused body. The mouth parts are part of an anterior structure known as a **capitulum,** which should be grasped firmly with forceps when removing an embedded tick to avoid leaving mouth parts in the skin. The thorax is fused to a globular body; head and antennae are absent. The adults have four pairs of legs. Acarid families include the following:

1. **Ixodidae**—a family containing the hard ticks that are temporary ectoparasites that feed on the host during larval, nymphal, and adult stages. Eggs are laid in the environment. Ticks can transmit several bacterial, rickettsial, viral, and at least one protozoan organism to humans, as noted in Table 6–1. Humans become infected with various organisms when the tick is feeding. Usually the pathogen enters the blood stream directly, but may also be rubbed into a wound if the area around the wound is contaminated with tick feces. An infected tick that has been crushed while removing it from people or pets may provide an additional source of infection. Furthermore, salivary secretions of some tick species can produce a toxemia (tick paralysis) which may result in death if the tick is not removed in time. And finally, bite wounds may become infected if mouth parts are left behind following tick removal. Ticks remain attached for extended feeding periods (up to several hours), and the local skin reaction to the mouth parts and the tick's salivary secretions becomes inflammatory and is often accompanied by edema and hemorrhage.

    Adult ticks may live for 2 to 3 or more years and will feed on several hosts. This longevity, coupled with the fact that most tick-borne organisms may be transmitted vertically (trans-stadial and/or transovarial passage), makes them very good vectors of disease.

2. **Argasidae**—a family containing the soft ticks that are also temporary ectoparasites. The body of soft ticks is soft and leathery, because it lacks the **scutum** found on the dorsal surface of hard ticks. These do not feed on humans.

3. **Sarcoptidae**—a family containing mites that are permanent ectoparasites which live and reproduce in burrows in the skin. Mites are quite host specific and are usually transferred to new hosts in crowded quarters where personal hygiene is neglected. Mites that normally infest other hosts may occasionally be temporary parasites of humans or other animals. For example, in the southern United States, *Ornithonyssus bacoti,* a species of bird mite, will migrate into homes from bird nests located in the eaves of houses. These insects will attack cats, dogs, and humans, causing dermatitis, papules, vesicles, and even tissue necrosis at the bite site.

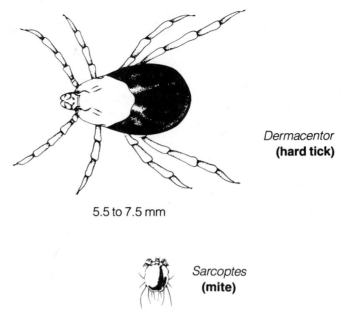

Dermacentor
(hard tick)

5.5 to 7.5 mm

Sarcoptes
(mite)

female 330 to 600 μm

The species *Sarcoptes scabiei* (the itch mite) causes the disease condition known as scabies (sarcoptic mange), which is diagnosed by finding the eggs, nymphs, or adults in skin scrapings of suspicious lesions. The diagnostic sign is a red tunnel measuring from a few millimeters to several centimeters in length which turns into an extremely itchy papule. These mites have a relatively short life cycle, and newly hatched larvae will reach adulthood in about 1 week. This short cycle allows infestations to become severe before treatment begins. *Sarcoptes scabiei* is endemic in the United States and elsewhere.

The morphologic characteristics of mites are similar to those seen in ticks except that mites do not have a scutum. They are microscopic in size, and their four pairs of legs are shorter, with only the two anterior pair extending past the margins of the body.

Treatment: 1 percent lindane or 10 percent crotamiton

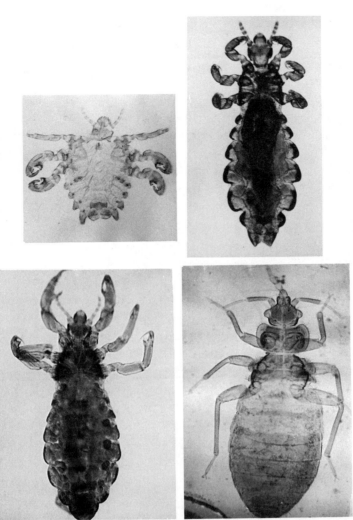
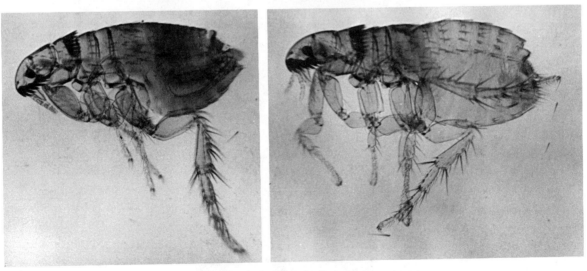

PHOTO 6–1 (top left). *Phthiris pubis* (crab louse), dorsal view (20×).

PHOTO 6–2 (top right). *Pediculus corporis* (body louse), dorsal view (15×).

PHOTO 6–3. (middle left). *Pediculus capitis* (head louse), dorsal view (20×).

PHOTO 6–4. (middle right). *Cimex lectularius* (bedbug), dorsal view (20×).

PHOTO 6–5 (bottom left). *Ctenocephalides* spp. (male dog or cat flea), lateral view (15×).

PHOTO 6–6 (bottom right). *Ctenocephalides* spp. (female dog or cat flea), lateral view (15×).

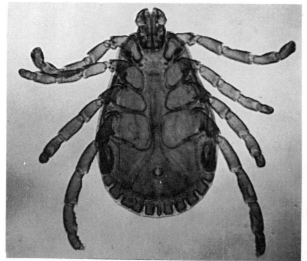

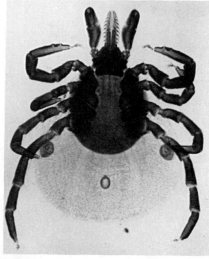

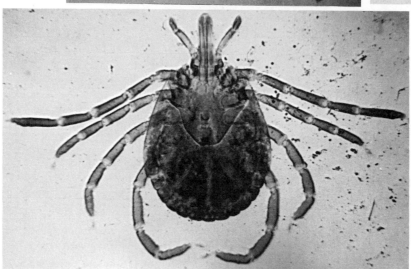

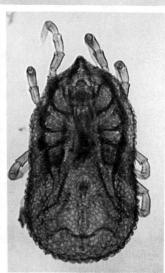

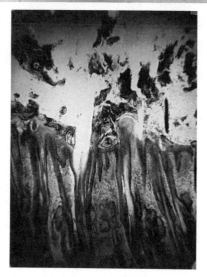

PHOTO 6–7 (top left). *Dermacenter andersoni* (hard tick), ventral view (10×).
PHOTO 6–8 (top right). *Ixodes* spp. (hard tick), dorsal view (20×).
PHOTO 6–9 (middle left). *Amblyomma americanum* (hard tick), dorsal view (10×).
PHOTO 6–10 (middle right). *Ornithodoros* spp. (soft tick), ventral view (10×).
PHOTO 6–11 (bottom). *Sarcoptes scabiei* (scabies in skin scraping) (40×).

TABLE 6–1. Arthropods of Medical Importance

Arthropod	Transmission Associations
Order Diptera (flies and mosquitoes) Families Culicidae (all mosquitoes)	
Aedes spp.	1. Viral—encephalitis, yellow fever, dengue fever, hemorrhagic fever 2. Nematoda—filariasis (*W. bancrofti*)
Anopheles spp.	1. Protozoa—malaria 2. Nematoda—filariasis (*W. bancrofti*—elephantiasis) (*B. malayi*) 3. Viral—various fevers and encephalitides
Culex spp.	1. Nematoda—filariasis (*W. bancrofti*) 2. Viral—encephalitis
Mansonia spp.	1. Nematoda—filariasis (*W. bancrofti*) (*B. malayi*) 2. Viral—various fevers
Family Ceratopogonidae (biting midges, punkies, no-see-ums)	
Culicoides spp.	1. Nematoda—filariasis (*M. ozzardi*) (*M. perstans*) (*M. streptocerca*)
Family Simulidae (black flies, buffalo gnats)	
Simulium spp.	1. Nematoda—filariasis (*O. volvulus*) (*M. ozzardi*)
Family Psychodidae (sand fly)	
Phlebotomus spp.	1. Protozoa—leishmaniasis (*Leishmania* spp.) 2. Viral—sand fly fever 3. Bacterial—*Bartonella bacilliformis*
Family Tabanidae (horse fly)	
Tabanus spp.	1. Bacterial—anthrax and tularemia (*B. anthracis*) (*F. tularensis*) 2. Protozoa—trypanosomes (mechanical transmission)
Chrysops spp. (mango fly) (deer fly)	1. Nematoda—filariasis (*Loa loa*)
Family Muscidae	
Musca spp. (house fly)	1. Bacterial—Tularemia (*F. tularensis*) 2. Mechanical vector of many protozoan species
Stomoxys spp. (stable fly)	1. Mechanical vector of many protozoan species

TABLE 6–1. *Continued*

Arthropod	Transmission Associations
Siphona spp. (horn fly)	1. Mechanical vector of many protozoan species
Glossina spp. (tsetse fly)	1. Mechanical vector of many protozoan species
	2. Protozoa—trypanosomiasis (*Trypanosoma* spp.)
Other Fly Families *Cochliomyia* spp.	1. Myiasis—primary and secondary—screwworm
Other genera	1. Myiasis—maggots (fly larvae on skin wound)—warbles (fly larvae inside tissues)
Order Hemiptera (bugs) **Family Reduviidae** *Triatoma* spp. *Rhodnius* spp. (kissing bugs)	1. Protozoa—visceral leishmaniasis (*T. cruzi*)
Family Cimicidae *Cimex* spp. (bedbug)	1. Itchy bites
Order Siphonaptera (fleas) **Family Pulicidae** *Xenopsylla* spp. (Oriental rat flea)	1. Bacterial—bubonic plague (black plague) (*Y. pestis*)
	2. Cestoda (*H. nana*) (*H. diminuta*)
	3. Rickettsial—murine typhus (*R. mooseri*)
Ctenocephalides spp. (cat or dog fleas)	1. Cestoda (*D. caninum*)
Order Parasitiformes **Family Ixodidae** (hard ticks) *Dermacentor* spp.	1. Rickettsial—Rocky Mountain spotted fever, Q fever (*R. rickettsii*) (*C. burnetti*)
	2. Bacterial—tularemia (*F. tularensis*)
	3. Viral—Colorado tick fever
Ixodes spp.	1. Protozoa—*Babesia* spp.
	2. Tick fever—*R. rickettsii*
	3. Viral—Colorado tick fever
	4. Spirochete (*Borrelia burgdorfia*)—Lyme disease

TABLE 6–1. *Continued*

Arthropod	Transmission Associations
Family Argasidae (soft ticks) *Ornithodoros* spp.	1. Bacterial—Relapsing fever (*Borrelia* spp.)
Family Sarcoptidae (mites) *Sarcoptes* spp. (mange mite)	1. Skin mange (*S. scabiei*)
Family Trombiculidae (mites) *Trombicula* spp. (chigger)	1. Rickettsial—scrub typhus (*R. tsutsugamushi*)
Order Anoplura (blood-sucking lice) Family Pediculidae *Pediculus* spp. (body lice)	1. Spirochetes—louse-borne relapsing fever (*B. recurrentis*) 2. Rickettsial—endemic typhus, trench fever (*R. prowazeki*) (*R. quintana*)
Phthirus pubis (crab louse)	1. Itchy bites
Order Mallophaga (biting lice) Family Trichodectidae *Trichodectes* spp. (biting lice of domestic mammals)	1. Cestoda—accidental infection (*D. caninum*) (*H. diminuta*)
Crustacea Order Copepoda *Cyclops* spp. (copepod) (water flea)	1. Nematoda—Guinea worm (*D. medinensis*) 2. Cestoda—fish tapeworm (*D. latum*) 3. Sparganosis—*Spirometra* spp.
Diaptomus spp. (copepod) (water flea)	1. Cestoda—fish tapeworm (*D. latum*)
Order Decapoda crayfish, crab	1. Trematoda—lung fluke (*P. westermani*)

You have now completed the section on Arthropoda. After reviewing this material with the aid of your learning objectives, proceed to the post-test.

BIBLIOGRAPHY

ALEXANDER, JOD: *Mites and skin diseases.* Clin Med 79:14, 1972.

BAKER, EW, ET AL: *A Manual of Parasitic Mites of Medical or Economic Importance.* National Pest Control Association Technical Publication, 1956.

BARNES, RD: *Invertebrate Zoology,* ed. 3. WB Saunders, Philadelphia, 1974.

BELDING, DL: *Textbook of Parasitology,* ed. 3. Appleton-Century-Crofts, New York, 1965.

BORROR, DJ, ET AL: *An Introduction to the Study of Insects,* ed. 4. Holt, Rinehart & Winston, New York, 1976.

BROWN, HW: *Basic Clinical Parasitology,* ed. 4. Appleton-Century-Crofts, New York, 1975.

DAVIES, JE, SMITH, RF, AND FREED, V: *Agromedical approach to pesticide management.* Ann Rev Entomol 23:353, 1978.

FAIN, A: *The Pentastomida parasitic in man.* Ann Soc Belg Med Trop 55:59, 1975.

FAUST, EC, BEAVER, PC, AND JUNG, RC: *Animal Agents and Vectors of Human Disease,* ed. 4. Lea & Febiger, Philadelphia, 1975.

Fleas of Public Health Importance and Their Control. CDC-DHEW Publication. U.S. Government Printing Office, Washington, DC, 1973.

HARVES, AD AND MILLIKAN, LE: *Current concepts of therapy and pathophysiology in arthropod bites and stings, Part 2. Insects: Review.* Int J Dermatol 14:621, 1975.

HOREN, PW: *Insect and scorpian stings.* JAMA 221:894, 1972.

Introduction to the Epidemiology of Vector-Borne Diseases. CDC-DHEW Publication, U.S. Government Printing Office, Washington, DC, 1960.

JAMES, MT: *The Flies That Cause Myiasis in Man.* Miscellaneous Publication No. 631, U.S. Government Printing Office, Washington, DC, 1947.

JAMES, MT AND HARWOOD, RF: *Hermes' Medical Entomology,* ed. 6. Macmillan, New York, 1969.

Lice of Public Health Importance and Their Control. CDC-DHEW Publication, U.S. Government Printing Office, Washington, DC, 1973.

ORKIN, J, MAIBACH, HI, PARISH, LC: *Scabies and Pediculosis.* JB Lippincott, Philadelphia, 1977.

Pest Control: An Assessment of Present and Alternative Technologies, Vol V. Pest Control and Health. Environmental Studies Board, National Research Council, National Academy of Science, Washington, DC, 1976.

SMART, J: *A Handbook for the Identification of Insects of Medical Importance.* British Museum, London, 1956.

SMITH, KGV (ED): *Insects and Other Arthropods of Medical Importance.* British Museum (Natural History), London, 1973.

STEERE, AC, BRODERICK, TF, AND MALAWISTA, SE: *Erythema chronicum migrans and Lyme arthritis: Epidemiologic evidence for a tick vector.* Am J Epidemiol 108:312, 1978.

Ticks of Public Health Importance and Their Control. CDC-DHEW Publication, U.S. Government Printing Office, Washington, D.C., 1974.

ZUMPT, F.: *Myiasis in Man and Animals in the Old World: A Textbook for Physicians, Veterinarians, and Zoologists.* Butterworth, London, 1965.

POST-TEST

1. Matching: enter the single best letter choice for parasite transmission: (**30 points**)

   a. ____ *Aedes*
   b. ____ *Anopheles*
   c. ____ *Simulium*
   d. ____ *Phlebotomus*
   e. ____ *Glossina*

   1. *Onchocerca volvulus*
   2. *Trypanosoma gambiense*
   3. *Leishmania donovani*
   4. *Giardia lamblia*
   5. *Brugia malayi*
   6. *Plasmodium vivax*

2. Indicate the type of Arthropoda that causes each of the following diseases or conditions. Use each letter as many times as appropriate. (**40 points**)

   a. ____ myiasis
   b. ____ blood loss
   c. ____ crabs
   d. ____ scabies
   e. ____ sleeping sickness
   f. ____ babesiosis
   g. ____ Rocky Mountain spotted fever
   h. ____ Chagas' disease
   i. ____ the black plague
   j. ____ malaria

   1. bug
   2. mosquito
   3. tick
   4. louse
   5. fly
   6. mite
   7. flea

3. Based upon your knowledge of the life cycle of fleas and lice, discuss control measures necessary to prevent the spread of each. (**10 points**)

4. State at least five ways in which Arthropoda are harmful to humans. (**20 points**)

7

CLINICAL LABORATORY PROCEDURES

LEARNING OBJECTIVES

Upon completion of this text and sufficient experience in a clinical parasitology laboratory, the student will be able to.

1. recognize potential sources of error in laboratory procedures.
2. recognize and sketch the important features of parasites present in clinical specimens which are routinely observed microscopically.
3. calibrate and correctly use an ocular micrometer to measure parasites.
4. demonstrate the proper technique of handling and disposing of contaminated materials.
5. state the proper procedures for collection and transport of fecal specimens.
6. select proper procedures for performing a routine fecal analysis for the presence of parasitic infections.
7. properly prepare fecal smears.
8. properly prepare iodine-stained and unstained wet mounts of fecal material.
9. correctly perform the trichrome stain on fecal material.
10. properly scan a microscope slide for the presence of parasites and identify by scientific name all parasites found therein.
11. select appropriate concentration technique for the recovery of any given parasite.
12. correctly perform the zinc sulfate flotation and the formalin-ether sedimentation concentration techniques for recovery of intestinal parasites.
13. correctly prepare thin and thick blood smears.
14. correctly perform the Giemsa staining technique for blood smears.
15. identify parasites in a stained blood sample.
16. select proper procedures and protocol for the identification of *Filaria* infections.
17. identify parasites present on a cellophane tape preparation for pinworms.
18. prepare and maintain *in vitro* cultures of protozoa.
19. correctly and accurately perform a fecal egg count.
20. prepare all solutions used routinely in the laboratory.
21. prepare serum for parasite serology.
22. correctly perform and evaluate serologic tests for parasitic infections.

FECAL EXAMINATION

General considerations for a routine fecal examination in the clinical laboratory include the following:.

1. Naturally passed stools are preferred for examination. Specimens can be passed into a clean wide-mouth cardboard container or bedpan. Samples collected in a bedpan **must not** be contaminated with urine and must be transferred to an appropriate container before submitting it to the laboratory. All specimens must be correctly and completely labeled. Protozoan cysts may be found more commonly in formed stools and are often easier to identify than trophozoites. Trophozoites are found more commonly in liquid stools or those obtained by saline purgation. Because trophozoites do not survive for great lengths of time and their motility is of diagnostic importance, specimens should be examined within 1 hour after passage. If transportation to the laboratory is to be delayed, part of the specimen should be immediately preserved in polyvinyl alcohol fixative (PVA-fixative)* or in 10 percent aqueous formalin.* Formalin preserves eggs, cysts, and larvae for wet-mount examination and for concentration. PVA-fixative preserves cysts and trophozoites for permanent staining.

2. Formed stools may be refrigerated for 1 to 2 days if their examination must be delayed, although this practice does not guarantee the recovery of all parasites. If examination must be delayed more than 4 hours, the specimen should be preserved in PVA or formalin. (Hookworm eggs mature and hatch if allowed to remain at room temperature and may be confused with *Strongyloides* larvae unless carefully observed.) (See also page 132 for transport procedures).

3. One or two specimens should be sufficient for the recovery and identification of helminth eggs.

4. When amebiasis or giardiasis is suspected, several specimens (at least three) should be examined, one every other day. Additional specimens are examined when necessary. For each specimen received, a permanently stained slide should be prepared and examined. Purged specimens must be examined immediately, or they are worthless. Saline purges using Epsom salt, sodium sulfate, or Fleet's Phospho-Soda are satisfactory, but castor and mineral oils make examination for protozoa impossible.

5. Feces containing x-ray contrast media, such as barium salts, are to be rejected, because these make a proper examination impossible.

6. Culture media for growth of *Entamoeba histolytica,* such as Balamuth's, Boeck and Drbohlav's, McQuay's, or Cleveland-Collier's media, may be useful. Various authorities express conflicting views on the relative usefulness of culture media, inasmuch as the number of cysts needed for viable cultures may be so great that they should be detectable at that number in feces by ordinary microscopic methods.

7. Care should be taken to maintain all working space in a neat and clean condition. All contaminated materials should immediately be placed in a disinfectant. Spills should be overlayed with a 50:50 solution of xylene and 70 percent alcohol prior to clean-up. (This will kill all protozoa and eggs, including *Ascaris.*) Rubber gloves and a protective coat or apron should be worn when handling feces. Nothing should be placed in the mouth when in the laboratory.

---

*Methods of preparation of reagents marked by asterisks are described on pages 138–140.

MACROSCOPIC EXAMINATION

The process of macroscopic examination, a routine component of a fecal examination for parasites, involves the following procedures:

1. Note the consistency of the specimen. Mushy or liquid stools suggest the possible presence of trophozoites or intestinal protozoa. Protozoan cysts are found more frequently in formed stools. Helminth eggs and larvae may be found in either liquid or formed stools.
2. Examine the surface of the specimen for parasites (e.g., tapeworm proglottids or, less commonly, adult pinworms).
3. Break up the stool with applicator sticks to check for the presence of adult helminths (e.g., *Ascaris*).
4. Examine the stool for blood and/or mucus.
   a. Fresh blood (bright red) indicates acute lower intestinal tract bleeding.
   b. Bloody mucus suggests ulceration, and some of this material should be preferentially examined microscopically for trophozoites.
5. Feces should be sieved after drug treatment for tapeworms to assure recovery of the scolex.

Of Note

1. Adult worms, if recovered, are examined and identified directly.
2. Tapeworms are speciated by examining gravid proglottids. Because eggs of *T. solium* are infective for humans, great care must be exercised when handling these specimens.
3. When examining a gravid proglottid, it should be fixed in 10 percent formalin and then cleared by immersing it in glycerin or lactophenol solution (1:1). Uterine branches may be made more visible by injecting a small amount of India ink into the uterine pore. A 1-ml syringe with a 26-gauge needle should be used to inject the ink. The segment should then be flattened by gently pressing it between two glass slides.

MICROSCOPIC EXAMINATION

Considerations to be observed in microscopic examination are given below.

DIAGRAM 7–1.

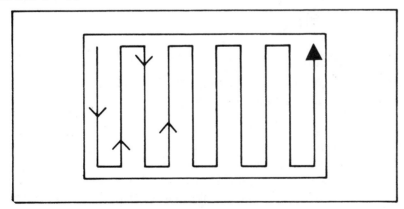

1. Any parasites detected are reported by their scientific name.
2. Direct wet mounts are prepared by using an applicator stick to thoroughly mix a small amount of feces with a drop of saline placed on a microscope slide. Apply a 22-mm cover glass so that air bubbles are not trapped under the glass. A smear should be thin enough so that a printed page can be read through it. The entire preparation must be examined for the presence of eggs, larvae, and protozoa.

Systematic examination, using the 10× lens, may be accomplished by starting at the lower edge of the slide and observing each field until the upper edge is reached (Diagram 7–1). Then move the preparation one field to the right and examine each field downward until the lower edge is reached. Move right one field and continue in this manner until the entire slide has been examined. Next, several random fields should be examined using the high dry objective lens, inasmuch as protozoa may have been overlooked at 10× magnification. Care must be exercised when adjusting the light on the microscope. A common error is the use of too much light, which prevents proper contrast. Because protozoa are translucent and colorless when unstained, they will not be visible unless the light is reduced. Iodine* may be used to help demonstrate eggs and cyst structures more clearly, but this kills and distorts trophozoites so that motility cannot be observed. A saline mount and an iodine mount may be prepared at opposite ends of the same slide, using separate cover slips.

DIAGRAM 7–2.

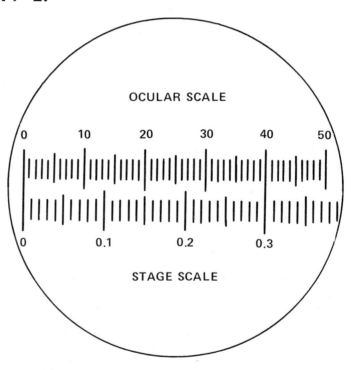

OCULAR SCALE

0   10   20   30   40   50

0   0.1   0.2   0.3

STAGE SCALE

3. A calibrated ocular micrometer should be employed routinely. Size differences of various internal structures and of whole organisms is important in differential diagnosis.
   a. Install an ocular micrometer disk in the eyepiece of the microscope by placing it underneath the eyepiece lens.
   b. Place a stage micrometer on the microscope's stage, and using the 10× objective, focus on the stage scale. The stage scale is one millimeter long and is calibrated in hundredths; each .01 mm = 10 microns.
   c. Line up the left edge of the ocular scale with the left edge of the stage scale (Diagram 7–2).
   d. Find a place at the farthest point to the right where a line on the ocular micrometer is exactly superimposed on a line of the stage micrometer.
   e. The number of microns indicated by each division on the ocular scale can be calculated using the following formula:

$$\frac{\text{Number of stage micrometer spaces} \times 10 \text{ microns}}{\text{Number of ocular micrometer spaces}} = \text{microns/ocular space}$$

Example: In Diagram 7–2, note that the fortieth ocular space is exactly superimposed with the thirtieth stage space (0.3 mm). Using the formula: $30 \times 10/40 = 7.5$ microns/ocular space.

   f. Steps two through six must be repeated for each objective lens. Record the calibration equivalent for each objective so that parasites may be measured when viewed at any magnification.

   g. To measure a parasite, line up one edge of the egg or cyst with the zero on the ocular scale, count the number of ocular spaces to the other edge, and multiply by the appropriate lens factor (e.g., $\times$ 7.5 microns in the example above).

CONCENTRATION TECHNIQUES FOR PARASITE STAGES IN FECES

A fecal concentration technique increases the possibility of detecting parasites when few are present in feces and is a routine part of the clinical procedures. A single concentrate from one fecal specimen is frequently sufficient to detect clinically important infections.

Two general types of methods are used—sedimentation and flotation. The formalin-ether sedimentation concentration method of Ritchie is the most commonly used technique for concentrating eggs and cysts and is more efficient than flotation methods.

SEDIMENTATION METHOD
Procedure for the Formalin-Ether* Method

This method concentrates parasite stages present in a large amount of feces into about 2 gm of sediment.

1. 10 to 20 gm (about 1 teaspoon) of feces is crushed with applicator sticks and mixed well with 10 to 12 ml of saline. The mixture is then filtered through two layers of dampened surgical gauze into a 15-ml conical centrifuge tube.
2. The suspension is centrifuged at 500 $\times$ g (1800 rpm)† for 5 minutes. The supernatant is decanted into disinfectant. The sediment is resuspended and recentrifuged in saline if there is excessive debris in the sample.
3. The washed stool sediment is suspended in 10 ml of 10 percent formalin and allowed to stand 5 minutes. This step kills and preserves protozoa, larvae, and most eggs. (Some eggshells, such as *Ascaris*, are impervious to formalin.)
4. 3 ml of ether* are added, the tube stoppered,* inverted, shaken vigorously for 10 seconds, and then centrifuged for 2 minutes at 1500 rpm. (This step extracts fats from the feces and reduces bulk.) Remove stopper carefully away from the face as ether vapor may cause spurting of fecal debris.
5. After rimming the upper debris layer with an applicator stick (Diagram 7–3), the entire supernatant is decanted into disinfectant. Invert the centrifuge tube completely in one smooth motion, but only one time. A small drop of fecal sediment and one drop of iodine stain are then mixed together on a slide. A cover glass is added, and the entire preparation is examined carefully for parasites. An unstained preparation also should be examined, since cysts are refractile and more easily detected unstained and morphology of larval forms will be more characteristic.

Of Note

1. Ethyl acetate may be substituted for ether in Step 4. Ethyl acetate is nonflammable and therefore is a much safer chemical for laboratory use. Recovery of *Hymenolepis nana* eggs and cysts of *Giardia lamblia* is enhanced with this reagent.

---

*Make certain there are no open flames in the room when ether is being used as it is highly combustible; be certain tubes and stoppers to be used are not soluble in ether.

†rpms are noted so that workers may more easily adjust speeds to the appropriate gravity when using common table-top centrifuges.

DIAGRAM 7–3.

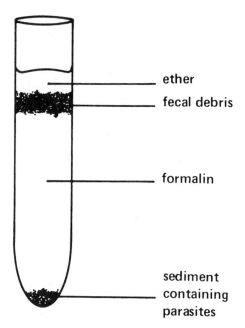

ether

fecal debris

formalin

sediment
containing
parasites

2. The sedimentation procedure can be used to concentrate PVA-fixed material as follows: thoroughly mix the PVA-stool suspension with applicator stick; add about 4 ml of the mixture to a test tube containing 10 ml of saline and mix well; filter the mixture through gauze as in Step 1 and continue the procedure as above. Extra washing of the sediment may be necessary, since iodine will cause precipitation of excess mercuric chloride. If precipitation is noted when the slide is examined, simply re-wash the sediment once or twice and prepare a new slide. Some authorities do not recommend concentrating PVA-fixed material, since protozoa are so distorted that they are not recognizable.

FLOTATION METHODS

Flotation methods use liquids with a higher specific gravity than that of eggs or cysts, so that parasites will float to the surface and can then be skimmed from the top of the tube. The concentrating solution should have a final specific gravity of about 1.20. The most commonly used reagent is zinc sulfate, and the procedure using this solution is described below. It is important to note that operculated eggs as well as schistosome and infertile ascaris eggs are not easily recovered by this method. In addition, the high specific gravity kills trophozoites and causes distortion of certain other fragile eggs, such as *Hymenolepis nana*. For these reasons, it is recommended that if only a single concentration procedure is being used, it should be the formalin-ether sedimentation technique.

Procedure for the Zinc Sulfate* Flotation Method

1. Prepare washed feces in a 13 × 100 mm round bottom tube as described in Steps 1 and 2 of the procedure for the formalin-ether method.
2. Resuspend and thoroughly mix the sediment in 12 ml of zinc sulfate solution (specific gravity, 1.18 to 1.20, as verified with a hydrometer).
3. Centrifuge for 1 minute at 650 × g (2000 rpm). Place tube in a rack in a vertical position and slowly add enough zinc sulfate with a dropper pipette to fill the tube so that an inverted meniscus forms (Diagram 7–4).
4. Without shaking the tube, carefully place a 22 × 22 mm cover glass on top of the tube so that its underside rests on the meniscus. The meniscus should not be so high that fluid runs down the side of the tube carrying parasitic forms away from the cover glass.

DIAGRAM 7–4.

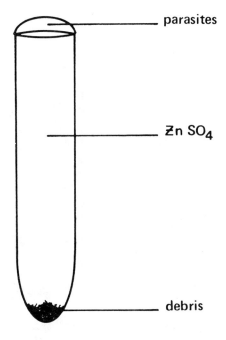

parasites

Zn SO$_4$

debris

5. Allow the tube to stand vertically in a rack with the coverslip suspended on top for 10 minutes.
6. Carefully lift the cover glass with its hanging drop containing parasites on the underside and mount on a clean slide, liquid side down. A small drop of iodine stain may be placed on the slide prior to adding the cover glass. The slide is gently rotated after adding the cover glass to insure a uniform mixture. The coverslip preparation is thoroughly examined microscopically, using the procedure outlined on page 125.

Of Note
Because gravity flotation is not particularly effective in concentrating organisms, many workers prefer the following variation:

1. After washing as in Step 1, resuspend sediment in 12 ml of zinc sulfate solution. Then fill the tube to within 0.5 ml of its top.
2. Centrifuge for 1 to 2 minutes at 500 × g (1800 rpm) and allow the centrifuge to stop without interference.
3. Carefully remove the tube from the centrifuge without shaking, and use a wire loop (bent at a right angle to the stem) to transfer 2 or 3 loopfuls of the surface film to a clean glass slide. Add a drop of iodine stain, mix, and add a cover glass. Examine microscopically.
4. Öocysts of *Isospora belli* and some other organisms are so lightweight that they will float very near the top of the liquid. It is important not to allow liquid to run down the side of the tube when placing a coverslip on top of the tube in Step 1 above. Also, and for the same reason, it is important to skim the top of the meniscus when using a wire loop as mentioned above.

CELLOPHANE TAPE TEST FOR PINWORM

As the female pinworm (*Enterobius vermicularis*) migrates out of the anus to deposit her eggs on the perianal region, eggs may be easily recovered there for identification. A parent can collect the specimen from a young child at home using a kit supplied by the doctor.

DIAGRAM 7–5.

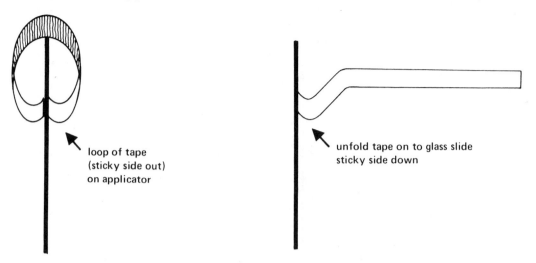

loop of tape
(sticky side out)
on applicator

unfold tape on to glass slide
sticky side down

Procedure

The following test should be done in the morning before the patient has washed or defecated, since the eggs are generally deposited in the perianal region at night.

1. Fold the edges of a 3 × ¾ inch piece of clear cellophane tape around the end of a tongue depressor so that the sticky side is out.
2. Spread the buttocks and apply the tape face to the anal area, using a rocking motion to cover as much of the perianal mucosa as possible.
3. Remove the tape and apply it to a microscope slide, sticky side down. Press firmly so that no air bubbles are trapped (Diagram 7–5).
4. Examine the slide for pinworm eggs under low power, using low light as described in the microscopic examination on page 125. Be sure to examine the entire area under the tape. The eggs are colorless; therefore, good focus and low light contrast are critical.

Of Note

1. Pinworm infection should not be ruled out until at least five daily consecutive negative preparations have been examined.
2. Cellulose tape can be cleared by lifting one edge of the tape from the slide and then place 1 or 2 drops of xylol or tolulol under the tape before examination. Disperse the liquid by carefully pressing the tape down onto the slide.

STOLL'S EGG-COUNTING TECHNIQUE

After a parasite has been identified, it may be necessary to determine the intensity of the infection. Parasitic disease pathology usually correlates with the number of worms present. Daily egg outputs of the various helminth species are known. Estimates of the worm burdens are accomplished, therefore, by counting the number of eggs found in a known amount of feces and calculating the number of worms required to produce this many eggs. Many variables, such as diet, faulty digestion, cycles of egg production, and the consistency of the stool, influence the results, but counts performed before and during treatment may guide the course of therapy, and those done afterward will monitor its success. The best results are achieved when counts are done on succeeding specimens obtained over a period of several days so that the average daily egg output may be determined.

Procedure

1. Fill a 100-ml graduated cylinder to the 56-ml mark with 0.1 N sodium hydroxide.
2. Using applicator sticks, add enough feces to raise the fluid level to the 60-ml mark.
3. Add 10 small glass beads, stopper tightly, and shake until the feces are completely broken up. Hard stools may need to sit in the NaOH for several hours or overnight in the refrigerator to become soft.
4. When the feces are completely dissolved, shake for 1 minute and immediately remove 0.075 ml of suspension and place it on a glass slide 1½ × 3 inches. Add a 22-mm square cover glass.
5. Use 100× magnification and count all eggs in the whole preparation. Be sure to look for eggs in any liquid around the edge of the cover glass.
6. Perform two counts using separate aliquots of 0.075 ml of suspension (total = 0.15 ml).

Calculation

1. The original fecal dilution is 1 to 15 (4 ml/60 ml). Since eggs in a total volume of 0.15 ml were counted, the total number of eggs in 1 ml of feces is found by multiplying the total count by 100 ($1/15 \times 0.15 \times 100 = 1$).
2. Assuming that the average person passes 100 gm of feces per day, it is possible to calculate the number of eggs per day by multiplying the answer by 100 (or the original suspension count by 10,000).
3. To determine the number of female worms present, divide the number of eggs present in feces per day by the average number of eggs produced by one female per day.

> Female *Necator* spp.—7000 eggs/day
> Female *Ascaris* spp.—200,000 eggs/day
> Female *Trichuris* spp.—7500 eggs/day

4. Total worm burden is found by multiplying the answer found in Step 3 by two, because it is assumed that random infections provide one male worm for every female worm.
5. Some workers believe that correction factors for stool consistency must be used to obtain accurate results. To do this, the number obtained in Step 1 should be multiplied by the appropriate factor. Formed stools = 1, mushy-formed = 1.5, mushy-diarrheic = 3, flowing diarrheic = 4, and watery = 5.

Of Note

1. A somewhat more accurate count may be obtained if a 24-hour stool collection is saved and weighed. Exactly 4 gm of mixed feces is then used in Step 1 of the counting procedure.
2. The calculation in Step 1 then is reported as eggs/gm of feces. This result may be multiplied by the total gm weight of the 24-hour specimen to give the total egg count/24 hours.
3. Clinically significant egg counts are as follows:
   a. *Necator* spp.—3000–12,000 eggs/gm of feces indicate the presence of about 70 to 350 worms and is associated with moderate infections.
   b. *Ancylostoma* spp.—6000–15,000 eggs/gm of feces indicate the presence of about 70 to 350 worms, since this parasite produces about twice as many eggs/day as *Necator* spp.
   c. *Ascaris* spp.—More than 16,000 eggs/gm of feces indicate the presence of at least 16 worms. Although infections of less than about 12 worms is usually asymptomatic, even one worm may cause symptoms if, for example, it invades the bile duct.

d. *Trichuris* spp.—30,000 eggs/gm of feces indicate the presence of about 600 worms and is associated with symptomatic infections. Less than 10,000 eggs/gm of feces are associated with asymptomatic infections.

SPECIMEN TRANSPORT PROCEDURES

Many laboratories in small hospitals, private clinics, or physicians' offices do not routinely perform examinations for eggs and parasites. These laboratories must send specimens to larger laboratories. Successful diagnosis of intestinal parasitic diseases requires "fresh" stool specimens. When examinations must be delayed, it is important to preserve specimen integrity by placing it in a proper transport medium.

A two-vial system is currently accepted as a standard means for transport. One vial should contain 8 to 10 ml of polyvinyl alcohol (PVA) fixative,* and a second vial should contain 8 to 10 ml of 10 percent formalin.* To each vial, 2 to 3 ml of feces is added. Be sure to select appropriate (e.g., bloody, slimy, or watery) areas. Sample material should be taken from the outer edge, ends, and middle of formed stools. Thoroughly mix the sample using applicator sticks. Cap the vial tightly. The specimen is now ready for transport. Additionally, a 2-ml sample of feces may be placed in a clean empty vial so that other examinations such as amoeba culture or the rearing of hookworm larva may be performed.

The receiving laboratory will then process the sample. Smears for trichrome* staining should be made from the PVA tube. Direct wet mounts made from the 10 percent formalin vial can be examined, and either tube may be used as source material for the formalin-ether concentration method. The zinc sulfate flotation method can be performed using the 10 percent formalin vial.

TRICHROME* STAIN FOR INTESTINAL PROTOZOA

The trichrome technique is a rapid procedure giving good results for routine identification of intestinal protozoa in fresh fecal specimens. The cytoplasm of *E. histolytica* trophozoites and cysts appears light blue-green or light pink. *E. coli* cysts are slightly more purple. Nuclear structure is clearly visible; karyosomes of nuclei stain ruby red. Degenerated organisms stain pale green. Background material stains green, providing a good contrast with the protozoa. The procedure requires that fecal smears be fixed with either PVA* or Schaudinn's* solution.

1. Using an applicator stick, place a thin film of fresh feces on a microscope slide, and while wet, place the smear in Schaudinn's fixative (without acetic acid) for 5 minutes at 50°C or 1 hour at room temperature. (Omit this fixation if smears have been preserved in PVA.) Diarrheic stools should be mixed with PVA-fixative. The fixative acts as an adhesive. When using PVA-fixed material from a transport vial, the following procedure should be followed:
   a. Pour some of the fecal material preserved in PVA onto a paper towel. Allow it to stand for 3 minutes. This step absorbs excess PVA solution and will improve staining results. This must be done on a surface that can be satisfactorily disinfected and the soiled toweling disposed of properly. An autoclavable tray may do.
   b. Using an applicator stick, spread some of the specimen from the towel onto a clean glass slide. Adherence to the slide is improved if the material is spread to the edges of the slide.
   c. Slides should be dried overnight at room temperature or for several hours on a slide warmer or in a 37°C incubator. Morphologic distortion may result if slides are dried too rapidly. The slide must be dried thoroughly to avoid washing off the film during staining.
2. Place slide in the 70 percent ethyl alcohol solution (with enough iodine added to turn the alcohol the color of strong tea) for 2 minutes (10 minutes for PVA-fixed smears).

3. Place slide successively in two changes of 70 percent solutions of ethanol for 1 minute in each solution. Rinse gently in tapwater.
4. Place in trichrome* stain for 2 to 8 minutes.
5. Rinse in acidified 90 percent ethanol* for 10 to 20 seconds. Usually a brief dip in and out is sufficient.
   NOTE: Inasmuch as the acid alcohol continues to de-stain as long as it is in contact with the material, the time allowed should include the few seconds between the time the slide is removed from the de-stain and the subsequent rinse in 95 percent alcohol in Step 6.
6. Rinse quickly in two changes of 95 percent ethanol and place in absolute alcohol 1 minute.
   For more effective removal of the acid de-stain, two 95 percent alcohol washes are suggested instead of one. These should be changed frequently to prevent them from becoming so acid that the de-staining process will continue. Prolonged de-staining in acid alcohol (over 20 seconds) may cause the organisms to be poorly differentiated. Larger trophozoites, particularly those of *E. coli,* may, however, require slightly longer periods of decolorization.
   NOTE: If several slides are being stained simultaneously, they should be de-stained separately. Remove only one slide at a time from the stain, de-stain it, rinse in the 95 percent alcohols, and place it in xylene (Step 7).
7. Place in xylene for 5 minutes.
8. Mount with a cover glass, using balsam or another mounting medium.
9. Examine under oil immersion as described previously.

NOTE: Quality control for this procedure may be accomplished by obtaining white blood cells from a buffy cell layer of centrifuged blood, which is then added to parasite-negative fecal material. From this mixture smears are made and stained along with unknown slides. Known negative slides should be processed with each set of unknowns. Since trichrome stains are quite stable, it is usually only necessary to check each new batch of stain. If staining is done very infrequently, it is advisable that periodic checks be done—at least monthly. If positive fecal material is available from patients or quality control survey samples, control slides may be made from PVA-fixed material. Check white blood cells and known parasites for color.

PROTOZOA CULTURE MEDIA

Routine diagnosis of protozoan infections is usually possible without employing culture methods; however, several media are available that support growth of many protozoan species. Commonly used media for intestinal protozoa are either a semisolid base set up as slant tubes with a liquid overlay (Boeck and Drbohlav, Cleveland and Collier,[†] and McQuay's diphasic charcoal medium), or a nutritive fluid (Balamuth). The axenic culture medium of Diamond is a useful diphasic medium in which a chick embryo extract is used as a liquid overlay for a slanted nutrient agar base. Diamond's medium is a medium primarily used in research centers and is most useful when stock cultures of *Entamoeba histolytica* must be maintained. Details for the in-house preparation of these basic media may be found in the references cited in this chapter. Regardless of the medium chosen, careful handling of the culture is important in order to obtain successful results. Only fresh fecal specimens (less than 6 hours old) should be used, and at least two wet mounts made from the sediment should be examined after incubation, inasmuch as growth is slow and numbers may be few.

Procedure for Use

1. To any of the prepared media listed above, add a 5-mm loop of sterile rice powder.[‡]

[†]Available as Bacto Entamoeba Medium, Difco Laboratories, Detroit, Michigan.
[‡]Available from Difco Laboratories, Detroit, Michigan.

2. Add about 1.5 ml of fluid or semifluid feces to each tube used, or, if the stool is formed, add a pea-size portion to the tube and mix gently.
3. Incubate at 37°C for 24 hours, examine at least 0.1 ml of the surface of the semisolid sediment for trophozoites. PVA-fixed smears may be made from the surface material and stained with trichrome if desired.
4. All cultures not showing trophozoites should be transferred to new media by transferring the top half of the sediment to a tube containing fresh media, and the new tube is then incubated at 37°C for 24 hours after which the culture surface is examined as in Step 3. No further transfers are needed. The culture is considered negative at this point if parasites are not recovered.
5. To culture leishmania and *Trypanosoma cruzi*, use Novy-MacNeal-Nicolle (NNN)* medium at room temperature. Thirty percent defibrinated rabbit blood in the agar and antibiotics in the fluid overlay are preferred. Aspirate material, bone marrow, chancre, or blood may be used as culture specimens. Check condensate at the bottom of the slant for 1 month for the presence of organisms.

BLOOD SMEAR PREPARATION AND STAINING FOR BLOOD PARASITES

These procedures are used for the recovery and identification of malaria, trypanosomes, microfilaria, and other parasites found in blood. Both thin and thick smears should be prepared, stained, and examined. Thin smears offer the advantage of very little distortion of the parasite, but the disadvantage is that many fields must be examined in order to detect parasites when they are few in number. While thick smear preparations often distort the parasite's morphology, the chances of detecting parasites are improved. Because this technique concentrates blood, the same volume of blood can be screened about three times faster than that in a thin smear. If improperly made, however, thick smears are useless.

DIAGRAM 7–6.

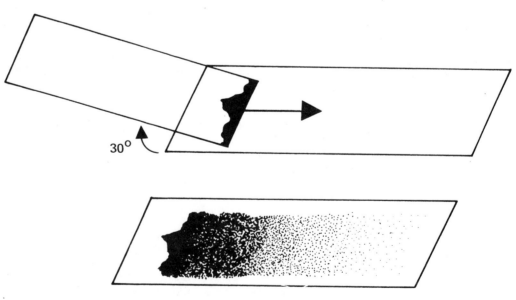

30°

SMEAR PREPARATION

Thin smears are prepared by touching a clean grease-free slide to a small drop of blood so that the drop is near one end of the slide. A second spreader slide is held on edge at a 30-degree angle on the slide holding the specimen and drawn back into the drop, allowing it to spread along the edge of the spreader slide (Diagram 7–6). Then, smoothly and rapidly, push the spreader slide forward so that the blood spreads out and trails in a flat sheet. The amount of blood should be small enough so that it is all spread before the spreader reaches the end of the specimen slide. Allow to air dry and stain as described. Screen the thin film for 30 minutes under 100× and also examine 100 to 200 microscopic fields of the thick film under oil immersion before reporting a specimen as negative.

Thick smears are prepared by touching a clean slide to a drop of blood. Using a corner of another slide, spread the blood evenly in a circular film about 15 mm in diameter. Allow to air dry overnight, and lake the blood by placing the slide in distilled water. (Laking may be omitted if a 1:50 Giemsa stain is used.) Laking causes RBCs to break open (i.e., lyse), causing hemoglobin's red color to disappear from the blood spot. Stain the laked blood smear as described below.

If filariasis is suspected, draw both diurnal and nocturnal blood samples to account for the periodicity of microfilaria. Perform a concentration test as described. In suspected malaria, if the first specimens are negative, retest the patient's blood every 6 hours for 1 full day to account for the periodicity of schizogony. Unstained and stained blood smears should be stored protected from insects and light in slide storage boxes. Quality control known positive and negative slides should be used routinely for all staining procedures on blood and feces.

GIEMSA* STAINING PROCEDURE

Thin smears: Fix the blood smear by immersing it in absolute methyl alcohol for 30 seconds. Place in working Giemsa stain (made by diluting stock Giemsa* 1:100 with pH 7.0 working buffer*) for 2 hours. The time may be reduced to 45 minutes if a 1:50 dilution is used, or 20 minutes if a 1:20 dilution is used. Rinse gently in buffer,* drain, and air dry. **(Do not blot.)** Examine under oil immersion as described above.

Thick smears: Place unlaked smears in a 1:50 dilution of stock Giemsa for 45 minutes. Wash gently with buffer for 2 minutes. Dry and examine under oil immersion.

(*Note:* New three-minute quick stains for blood smears are available. Each laboratory should carefully compare results with standard staining methods.)

KNOTT'S TECHNIQUE FOR CONCENTRATING MICROFILARIAE

When filariasis is suspected, it may be useful to concentrate blood in order to increase the possibility of finding microfilaria.

Procedure

1. Obtain 2 ml of whole blood by venipuncture and immediately place it in a centrifuge tube containing 10 ml of 2 percent formalin.
2. Stopper the tube and mix thoroughly by inverting and shaking the tube. The formalin lakes red blood cells, fixes blood protozoa, and kills and straightens the bodies of microfilariae.
3. Centrifuge the tube for 2 minutes at 500 × g (1800 rpm), or let it stand stoppered overnight in the refrigerator.
4. Decant the supernatant.
5. Remove the sediment with a Pasteur pipette and spread in a thick film on a slide.
6. The sediment may be examined wet for microfilariae, or the slide may be allowed to dry overnight, followed by staining with Giemsa for 45 minutes (see thick smear staining procedure above). De-stain in water (pH 7.2) for 10 to 15 minutes, allow to dry, and examine.

Ot Note

1. Although not routinely performed, it may be useful to examine fresh blood when trypanosomes or microfilariae are suspected. To perform this technique, one

needs only to place a drop of fresh blood on a slide, add a coverslip to prevent clotting, and examine under low power (10×) for microfilariae or high dry power (40×) for trypanosomes. Especially when parasites are few in number, they may be detected by their characteristic motility. The undulating motion of the trypanosome and the whiplike motion of the microfilariae are easily spotted as they cause movement of surrounding red blood cells and thus may shorten the examination time needed for a positive diagnosis.

2. Other concentration techniques are available, including filtering laked blood through a fine pore filter and then staining the filter for microfilariae; and passing blood through Sephadex filters, which selectively attach trypanosomes that can be later eluted. Stained blood films still must be examined in order to correctly identify the species of parasite.

SEROLOGIC METHODS

TABLE 7–1. Serodiagnostic Tests for Parasitic Diseases

PARASITIC DISEASES	Complement Fixation	Bentonite Flocculation	Indirect Hemagglutination	Latex	Special Tests	Indirect Immunofluorescence	Immunodiffusion	Immunoelectrophoresis	Countercurrent Electrophoresis	Enzyme Linked Immunoassay-Elisa	Radio Immunoassay	Detection of Circulating Antigen
African Trypanosomiasis	▲		▲			■	■			■		
Amebiasis	■	■	■	■	○A C	■	■	■	■	▲		○
Ancylostomiasis	○		■	▲		○		○				
Ascariasis	■	■	■			▲	▲	○		■	○	
Chagas	■		■	■	■A	■	○	▲	■	▲		○
Clonorchiasis	■		■			○	○	○				○
Cysticercosis	▲	▲	■	▲		▲	▲	○	○	○		
Echinococcosis	■	■	■	■		■	■	■	■	■	○	
Fascioliasis	■	○	■	▲		■	■	■	■	○		
Filariasis	▲	■	■	○		■		▲	▲	▲	○	▲
Giardiasis						▲	○			▲		
Leishmaniasis	■		■	■	■A	■	○	○	○	▲	○	
Malaria	▲		■	▲		■	■	○	▲	■	○	▲
Paragonimiasis	■	○	○			▲	▲	○	○			○
Pneumocystosis	■			○		■						▲
Schistosomiasis	■	■	■	○	■B C	■	▲	■	▲	■	○	■
Strongyloidiasis			■			▲				○		
Toxocariasis	○	■	■			▲	■	○		■	○	○
Toxoplasmosis	■		■	■	■C	■	○			■	○	▲
Trichinellosis	■	■	■	■		■	■	▲	■	■	○	○

○ Reported in literature   A Direct agglutination

▲ Experimental test   B COPT – circumoval precipitin test

■ Evaluated test   C FIAX™ automated fluoroimmunoassay

Courtesy of Dr. Irving Kagen, Centers for Disease Control, Parasitic Disease Division, Atlanta, Georgia

Serologic testing is becoming more useful in the diagnosis of parasitic diseases, particularly as commercial products become more readily available. Current methods include immunofluorescence tests; slide, tube, and agar precipitin tests; complement fixation; particle agglutination tests; and enzyme-linked immunoassays, among others (Table 7–1). These procedures are most useful for diseases that cannot be diagnosed by routine fecal or blood examination.

Since clinical manifestations of several parasitic diseases such as amebiasis of the liver, echinococcosis, trichinellosis, toxoplasmosis, and schistosomiasis are not always clear-cut, it is possible to help confirm the diagnosis of these diseases serologically, when the measurable antibody titer has reached a detectable level in serum. In the United States, serum for such studies is commonly sent for serologic testing to a State Public Health Reference Laboratory or to the Centers for Disease Control (CDC) in Atlanta, Georgia. Samples for CDC processing must be sent via state laboratories, as CDC will not accept specimens sent directly by laboratories or physicians. Most serum specimens may be shipped frozen or preserved with thimerosal (1:10,000 final concentration). The vial, containing at least 2 ml of serum, should indicate the preservative used. Serologic tests which have been performed are listed in Table 7–1. Table 7–2 lists the

TABLE 7–2. Immunodiagnostic Tests for the Diagnosis of Parasitic Diseases Performed by the Division of Parasitic Diseases, Center for Infectious Diseases, Centers for Disease Control

Diseases	Tests	Respective Diagnostic Titer(s)
Performed in protozoal diseases branch		
Amebiasis	IHA	≥1:256
Babesiosis	IIF	≥1:16
Chagas' Disease	CF; IIF	≥1:8, ≥1:16
Leishmaniasis	CF; IIF	≥1:8, ≥1:16
Toxoplasmosis	IIF; IIF-IgM; REIA	≥1:256; ≥1:64; ≥1:64
Performed in helminthic diseases branch		
Cysticercosis	ELISA; IMB	≥10%; positive
Echinococcosis	IHA; DD5	≥1:256; positive
Gnathostomiasis	IIF	Positive
Paragonimiasis	IMB	Positive
Schistosomiasis (mansoni)		≥10% activity units/μl
(japonicum &	ELISA	Positive
haematobium)	IMB	
Strongyloidiasis	IHA	≥1:128
Toxocariasis	ELISA	≥1:32
Trichinellosis	BFT	≥1:5
Performed in malaria branch		
Malaria	IIF	≥1:64

BFT: bentonite flocculation
CF: complement fixation
DD5: arc 5 double diffusion (done for specific confirmation)
ELISA: enzyme-linked immunosorbent assay
IHA: indirect hemagglutination
IIF: indirect immunofluorescence
IMB: immunoblot (Western blot)
REIA: reversed enzyme immunoassay
Courtesy of Dr. Lee Moore, Division of Parasitic Diseases, Centers for Disease Control, Atlanta, Georgia.
NOTE: See Table 7–3 for sources for some of the many commercial products available for use in immunodiagnosis in the laboratory.

types of tests for parasitic disease available at CDC. For state public health testing, consult locally. For more specific details about test procedures, the reader should consult the references found at the end of this chapter.

At this time, several companies offer reagents and supplies for individual laboratories that want to perform their own procedures. Table 7–3 includes procedures available from commercial suppliers. The list is not inclusive and in no way constitutes an endorsement by the authors of any product or supplier but is merely a resource guide for those interested in parasitic serology.

Errors in serologic diagnosis may be related to mixed infections, cross-reacting antigens shared with other parasites or other microorganisms, or even to nonparasite-related diseases, as well as to errors in technique. Quality-control tests using known positive and negative sera should always be performed.

TABLE 7–3. Commercial Serology Kits

Parasitic Disease	Test System	Supplier
African trypanosomiasis	Indirect Hemagglutination	1
Echinococcus granulosus	Indirect Hemagglutination	1,5
Entamoeba histolytica	Indirect Hemagglutination	1
	Agar Gel Dilution	2
	Countercurrent Electrophoresis	2
	Enzyme-labeled Immunoassay	2
Leishmaniasis	Indirect Hemagglutination	1
Schistosoma mansoni	Indirect Hemagglutination	1
Toxoplasma gondii	Indirect Hemagglutination	1,5
	Complement Fixation	1
	Enzyme-labeled Immunoassay	2
	Indirect Fluorescent Antibody	4
Trichinella spiralis	Agar Gel Diffusion	2
	Countercurrent Electrophoresis	2
	Enzyme-labeled Immunoassay	2
	Latex Agglutination	3,6

1. Behring Diagnostics (Calbiochem-Behring Corp.), 10933 North Torrey Pines Road, La-Jolla, CA 92037
2. Cordis Laboratories, P.O. Box 523580, Miami, FL 33152
3. Difco Laboratories, P.O. Box 1058A, Detroit, MI 38232
4. Microbiological Research Corp., Box 308, 40 West 500 South, Bountiful, UT 84010
5. Telcolab Corporation, Chrysler Building, 405 Lexington Avenue, New York, NY 10017
6. Wampole Laboratories, Cranbury, NJ 08512

REAGENT PREPARATION

D'ANTONI'S IODINE STAIN

1. Use when preparing wet-mount preparations of fresh or concentrated feces
2. Reagents
   a. 1 gm potassium iodine
   b. 1.5 gm powdered iodine crystals
   c. Add reagents to 100 ml of distilled water and shake well. Store in brown stoppered bottles; filter daily.

POLYVINYL ALCOHOL (PVA) FIXATIVE[†]

1. Use to preserve feces for transport or staining
2. Reagents
   a. ethyl alcohol, 95 percent   156 ml
   b. mercuric chloride, aqueous (saturated)   312 ml
   c. glacial acetic acid   25 ml
   d. PVA powder   20 ml
   e. glycerol   7.5 ml
   f. Mercuric chloride is prepared by dissolving 130 to 140 gm of the salt in 1000 ml of distilled water. Heat to dissolve, cool, filter, and store in a stock bottle.
   g. Add the PVA powder to the alcohol slowly, with stirring. Heat to 75°C and stir until the solution is clear. Add the other reagents and allow to cool. Store in a closed container and use as needed. Decant the solution without disturbing the sediment.
3. Between 2 and 3 ml feces per 8 to 10 ml PVA solution is adequate for transport. (Check government regulations on mailing.) Slides may be made from the transport vial. Polyvinyl alcohol also can be used by mixing one drop of fluid stool in three drops of PVA solution on a slide and allowing it to dry overnight at 37°C before staining.

10 PERCENT FORMALIN

1. Use with the formalin-ether sedimentation concentration method
2. Reagents
   a. formaldehyde   1 part
   b. physiologic saline   9 parts

ZINC SULFATE SOLUTION

1. Use with the zinc sulfate flotation concentration method
2. Reagents
   a. 330 gm zinc sulfate (reagent grade)
   b. distilled water (final volume—1 liter)
   c. Add reagent to the water with heat and stirring, and adjust the specific gravity to between 1.18 and 1.20, using a hydrometer

GIEMSA STAIN

1. Use to stain blood parasites
2. Reagents
   a. Giemsa stain may be purchased as a concentrated stock or stock Giemsa can be prepared as follows:
      (1) powdered Giemsa   1 gm
      (2) glycerol   66 ml
      (3) methanol (absolute)   66 ml
   b. Grind the stain in a mortar containing 5 to 10 ml glycerol. Add the remaining glycerol and heat to 55°C in a water bath until the stain is dissolved. Cool and add the methanol. Let stand for 2 to 3 weeks. Filter and store in a brown bottle away from light.
3. Before use, dilute with Giemsa buffer

GIEMSA BUFFER

1. Use with stock Geimsa stain
2. Reagents

[†]Bulk and prepackaged reagents are available from Meridian Diagnostics, Inc., Cincinnati, Ohio.

a. 0.067 M Na$_2$HPO$_4$ (disodium phosphate). Add 9.5 gm to 1000 ml of distilled water. This is stock buffer No. 1.
b. 0.067 M NaH$_2$PO$_4$ • H$_2$O (monosodium phosphate). Add 9.2 gm to 1000 ml of distilled water. This is stock buffer No. 2.
3. Working buffer, pH 7.0, is prepared from stock buffers weekly and filtered before use. To 900 ml distilled water add 61.1 ml of stock buffer No. 1 and 38.9 ml of stock buffer No. 2.

TRICHROME STAIN

1. Used to stain fecal smears for intestinal protozoa
2. Reagents
   a. Schaudinn's solution: Saturated aqueous mercuric chloride; 130 to 140 gm of mercuric chloride is added to 1000 ml of distilled water. Heat to dissolve, cool, then filter into a stock bottle. Working solution is prepared by mixing two parts of mercuric chloride solution with one part of 95 percent ethanol before use. Discard after use.
   b. Alcohol solutions: Various solutions may be prepared by diluting the appropriate volume of absolute (100 percent) ethanol with distilled water (e.g., a 70 percent solution is made by adding 30 ml of water to 70 ml of absolute alcohol). All alcohol solutions should be prepared fresh daily.
   c. Trichrome stain:

chromotrope 2R	0.6 gm
light green SF	0.15 gm
fast green FCF	0.15 gm
phosphotungstic acid	0.7 gm
acetic acid (glacial)	1.0 ml
distilled water	100 ml

   Mix the dry components and add the acetic acid; allow to stand for 30 minutes, then add to water. The stain should be purple. Staining over 14 smears daily tends to weaken the stain. Strength will return if the stain is exposed to air for 3 to 8 hours.

   Prepared trichrome stain, made by Remal, is available through major laboratory supply companies.
   d. Acid alcohol is prepared by adding one milliliter of acetic acid to 99 milliliters of 90 percent ethanol.

NNN MEDIUM

1. Use to culture blood, aspirates, bone marrow, biopsy, or other tissue material for *Leishmania* spp. and *Trypanosoma cruzi.*
2. Mix and bring to boiling the following ingredients:
   a. Agar: 14 g
   b. Sodium chloride: 6 g
   c. Distilled water: 900 ml
3. Distribute media to test tubes and sterilize in the autoclave.
4. Cool medium to 48°C and to each tube, add one third of its volume of sterilized defibrinated rabbit blood.
5. Mix thoroughly by rotation and allow to cool in a slanted position. Cooling is best done in an ice bath as rapid cooling promotes water condensation in the tube. Organisms develop most rapidly in the supernate at the bottom of the tube.
6. Check for sterility by incubating the medium overnight at 37°C.

You have now completed the section on clinical laboratory procedures. After reviewing this material with the aid of your learning objectives, proceed to the post-test.

BIBLIOGRAPHY

BEESON AND MCDERMOTT (EDS): *Cecil-Loeb Textbook of Medicine,* ed 13. WB Saunders, Philadelphia, 1971, pp 762–764.

BELDING, DL: *Textbook of Parasitology,* ed 3. Appleton-Century-Crofts, New York, 1965.

BROWN, HW: *Basic Clinical Parasitology,* ed. 4. Appleton-Century-Crofts, New York, 1975.

CHANDLER, AC AND READ, CP: *Introduction to Parasitology,* ed 10. John Wiley & Sons, New York, 1961, pp 402, 433.

CHITWOOD, M AND LICHTENFELS, JR: *Parasitological review. Identification of parasitic metazoa in tissue sections.* Exp Parasitol 32:407, 1972.

DIAMOND, LS: *Axenic culture of Entamoeba histolytica.* Science 134:336, 1961.

Difco Manual of Dehydrated Culture Media and Reagents for Microbiological and Clinical Laboratory Procedures, ed 9. Difco Laboratories, Detroit, 1953.

FAUST, EC, BEAVER, PC, AND JUNG, RC: *Animal Agents and Vectors of Human Disease,* ed 4. Lea & Febiger, Philadelphia, 1975.

FRANKEL, S, REITMAN, S, AND SONNENWIRTH, AC (EDS): *Gradwohl's Clinical Laboratory Methods and Diagnosis,* ed 7. CV Mosby, St. Louis, 1970, p. 1768.

GARCIA, LS AND ASH, LR: *Diagnostic Parasitology Clinical Laboratory Manual,* ed 2. CV Mosby, St. Louis, 1979.

GARCIA, LS AND BRUCKNER, DA: *Diagnostic Medical Parasitology.* Elsevier Science Publishers, New York, 1988.

KONEMAN, EW, RICHIE, LE, AND TIEMANN, C: *Practical Laboratory Parasitology.* Williams & Wilkins, Baltimore, 1974.

MACINNIS, AJ AND VOGE, M: *Experiments and Techniques in Parasitology.* WH Freeman, San Francisco, 1970.

MCQUAY, RM: *Charcoal medium for growth and maintenance of large and small races of Entamoeba histolytica.* Am J Clin Pathol 26(10):1137, 1956.

MELVIN, DM AND BROOKE, MM: *Laboratory Procedures for the Diagnosis of Intestinal Parasites.* U.S. Department of Health, Education and Welfare Publication (CDC)-75-82821, Atlanta, 1975.

MOST, H: *Drug therapy. Treatment of common parasitic infections of man encountered in the United States,* N Engl J Med 287:495, 1972.

WHEATLEY, WB: *A rapid staining procedure for intestinal amoebae and flagellates.* Am J Clin Path 2:990–991, 1951.

WYNGAARDEN, LB AND SMITH, LH: *Cecil Textbook of Medicine,* ed 16. WB Saunders, Philadelphia, 1982, p. 1766.

YOUNG, KH, ET AL: *Ethyl acetate as a substitute for diethyl ether in the formalin-ether sedimentation technique.* J Clin Microbiol 10:852–853, 1979.

POST-TEST

Mark True (T) or False (F) for each of the following: (*2 points each*)

_____ 1. In general, six sequential fecal specimens should be examined for the presence of any intestinal parasites.

_____ 2. Liquid or soft stools should be examined within 1 hour, since trophozoites die rapidly.

_____ 3. Formed stools need not be refrigerated, since protozoa have already formed cysts.

_____ 4. Wet mounts should be made when bloody mucus is noted in a stool specimen.

_____ 5. A castor oil enema may be used if only helminths are suspected.

_____ 6. It is not necessary to examine the whole slide if eggs or cysts are noted within the first few fields examined.

_____ 7. A careful examination of a stained thin smear of blood will reveal the presence of blood parasites.

Discussion questions: (**6 points each**)

8. How should the microscope's light be adjusted for successful microscopic examination of wet mounts and why?

9. When should a cellophane tape test be done and why?

10. Name two types of concentration methods, explain the principle, and write the procedure for each method named.

11. What is the specific gravity of the solution used in the zinc-sulfate concentration method? How is it checked?

12. Which eggs are not easily recovered by flotation methods?

13. What is used to extract fats in the sedimentation method?

14. List the advantages and disadvantages of thin and thick smears for blood parasites.

15. How is blood laked in the preparation of thick blood smears?

16. List the expected staining reactions for protozoa, using trichrome stain.

17. Name three protozoa culture media. What additional material is added to the culture at the time of inoculation?

18. Working Giemsa buffer is prepared from two stock solutions. What are the salts in each solution? What is the pH of the working buffer?

19. Match the reagents with the chemical components given: (**2 points each**)

a. _____ iodine crystals
b. _____ mercuric chloride
c. _____ rice powder
d. _____ light green SF
e. _____ monosodium phosphate
f. _____ phosphotungstic acid
g. _____ sugar
h. _____ 10% formalin
i. _____ 70% alcohol
j. _____ ether

1. PVA
2. D'Antoni's stain
3. Giemsa stain
4. Trichrome stain
5. Schaudinn's solution
6. Balamuth
7. sedimentation
8. flotation

CONTROL AND TREATMENT OF PARASITIC DISEASE

Most lay persons believe that treating an infected individual controls the parasitic disease and that avoiding an infected individual prevents catching the infection. These people also generally accept the idea that good hygienic practices lessen or prevent infections. Such concepts in fact do lead to a lower incidence of many diseases, but as you will see, the actual control of parasitic diseases in nature is far more complicated than this.

In order to control parasitic diseases adequately, we must give consideration to the parasite's life cycle, the cultural beliefs, personal hygiene, and dietary habits of the host as well as community affluence, education, sanitation, and medical practices. Further, local ecologic and biologic factors as well as the general health of local domestic and wild animals must enter the picture.

A parasite's life cycle may involve a single host with no free-living stages (such as *Enterobius*, which is very easily spread to others), whereas others have a very complex life cycle (such as *Clonorchis*) involving multiple hosts and parasite stages.

Control of pinworm infection, for example, relies heavily on preventing the contamination of bed linens by wearing nonporous close-fitting clothing to bed, by sterilizing sheets in boiling water, and by frequent vacuum cleaning of rugs and furniture. Also important is attention to details such as covering toothbrushes or other personal articles in order to guard against exposure to bathroom dust, which may carry airborne eggs. Sunlight (ultraviolet) will kill the larvae, as will dry heat; however, many household and other toxic chemicals will not penetrate the shell. Lack of cooperation between the patient and family members may actually hamper control and treatment.

Parasites such as *Schistosoma* which require an invertebrate host may be controlled by interrupting the life cycle; that is, by destroying the snail host itself or by destroying the infective cercaria larvae released into the water from the snail host. An advantage offered by this type of life cycle is that control measures do not depend heavily upon the involvement and the cooperation of the local citizenry but may be handled independently by knowledgeable experts in cooperation with the government.

Ensuring safe water and limiting the snail populations are the two most important and viable control measures for schistosomiasis. An example of such successful preventive management has occurred in Puerto Rico. Early in the control campaign, a trial mass chemotherapy treatment of infected individuals led to the death of some persons because of drug side effects. Chemotherapy was suspended and attention was focused on snail control. A molluscan competitor was introduced into ponds, lakes, and rivers in an effort to reduce the numbers of the specific host species. Concurrently, the project managers improved sanitary waste disposal systems, thus reducing the exposure of the snails to infective miracidium. By the mid-1960s, some 15 to 20 years of work began to show success. In most areas of Puerto Rico, the rate of infection in the population fell from 20 percent to almost zero.

Since schistosomiasis is still a major problem in many parts of the world, similar control methods are being tried elsewhere. However, another important control strategy is human behavior modification. Since human infections with schistosomiasis occurs when cercariae penetrate bare skin, something as simple as wearing wading boots when in water can break the parasite's life cycle. Shoes serve the same purpose in preventing hookworm and *Strongyloides* infections. Most important, by teaching people to use toilets or latrines, infected urine or feces do not contaminate soil or water supplies.

In controlling the spread of other parasitic diseases, chemical measures have had varying degrees of success. Remember—dormant stages of parasites, such as eggs and cysts, are generally resistant to toxic substances, which makes control of the environment difficult. A practical solution in many cases is vector control where an arthropod is involved. For instance, sprays and dips reduce flea and tick infestations in livestock and domestic pets even though it does not clear the environment. Biodegradable chemicals in water supplies have been used to control black fly larvae, and insecticide sprays are widely used to control the tsetse fly vector of trypanosomiasis.

The World Health Organization (WHO) sponsored an ambitious program to eradicate malaria worldwide. Early in the program, investigating members of the project found many mosquitoes resting inside houses. Consequently, they had the inside walls of houses and other buildings sprayed with DDT. This initially aggressive attack dramatically reduced the malaria problem in parts of Africa, but when local follow-up procedures became lax because of initial success, the incidence of malaria climbed dramatically. Some observers have claimed that the WHO program contributed greatly to the DDT resistance seen in mosquitoes, but the resistance problem can actually be traced to indiscriminate agricultural use of the chemical.

Another problem hampered WHO's African mosquito attack. Either two insect groups existed (house-dwelling and bush-dwelling), or some of the house-dwelling mosquitoes changed their behavior patterns and became bush-dwelling mosquitoes. Some investigators believed that the DDT house-spraying measures may have selected for the bush-dwelling mosquitoes. However, when the spraying stopped, the house-dwelling mosquitoes reappeared, suggesting still another biologic change. Regardless of the reasons for the changes, the DDT experience offers an example of the importance of understanding the complex biology and behavior patterns of insect vectors when choosing control strategies.

Of serious ecologic concern, however, is the past history of indiscriminant spraying of insecticide prior to human understanding of the biologic impact of chemicals such as DDT on all plants and animals in the food chain, as well as our failure to predict that such spraying would cause selection for insect vectors resistant to chemicals. These human errors should not be allowed to reoccur.

A more successful control experience occurred in Central America, where a well-planned strategy was used to control *Culicoides* spp., which bred in the Farfan Swamp in the Panama Canal Zone. These tiny biting gnats (no-see-ums) can fly through normal window screen mesh and forced workers caring for military communications equipment located in the swamp to wear finely meshed protective suits. Because temperatures often reached more than 90°F, the obvious discomforts forced other control measures to be sought. Chemical control of the insect in the swamp began in the early 1950s, but the gnat developed genetic resistance to the insecticide, making other control measures necessary.

The Farfan Swamp, although fed by a fresh water stream, was brackish because sea water backed up into it. Because the endemic *Culicoides* spp. breeds only in salty water, tidal gates were built to keep the sea water out of the swamp. Gradually, the swamp's water became fresh, and by the late 1950s, the gnat population had diminished to an acceptable level. Later in the mid-1960s, a canal dredging operation began dumping its dredge into the swamp, causing the water to become salty again. This change caused the gnat population to grow, and efforts were then made to halt dumping in the Farfan Swamp. It took about two years to clear the salt once again from the swamp water, and consequently, to bring the *Culicoides* back under control.

Various other methods of biologic insect and parasitic control have been tried. Elimination of primary screwworm fly myiasis from the southeastern United States was accomplished by releasing numerous male *Callitroga hominivorax* flies that had been sterilized by irradiation. Competitive mating decreased the offspring to below critical mass levels for breeding. Similar successful elimination in the southwestern United States has not been achieved because the insect population entering from Mexico could not be adequately controlled at the same time. By contrast, the Florida peninsula effectively isolated its area from invading flies. More recently, the state of California used irradiated flies in their campaign against the Mediterranean fruit fly. Daily, 20,000 irradiated flies raised in an agricultural research station in Hawaii were shipped to California. This helped save the fruit crop and lessened the need for chemical control measures. This example illustrates how combining various strategies can control insect populations.

Serious efforts are also being expended on perfecting other control systems. Immunization has already proven successful against several serious parasites of domestic animals. Other biologic methods are also being explored, such as improved insect traps using pheromones, genetic manipulation of insect hosts, introduction of predators for insect, snail, and other host species, introduction of competitive species of nonpathogenic parasites or nonsupportive hosts, and mass treatment of host populations with chemotherapeutic agents. For example, India, which spends 45 percent of its national health budget controlling malaria, is now looking to alternatives to the millions of dollars spent on pesticides. These include breeding fish in waters that harbor mosquito larvae and later selling the fish; filling in pits and creating usable land; and planting eucalyptus trees in swamps to soak up water and later using the wood for cooking and construction.

Cultural behavior of world populations both aids and hinders the control of parasitic diseases. For instance, the dietary customs of Jewish and Moslem peoples have greatly reduced their exposure to *Taenia solium* and *Trichinella spiralis* infections. On the other hand, people in many parts of the world, including the United States, still use untreated human waste (known as night soil) to fertilize crops. They also bathe and wash clothes and cooking utensils in water contaminated with human waste. Such behavior obviously promotes the transmission of parasites. In some wealthy countries, again including the United States, many people are getting back to nature or vacationing in health resorts offering natural or untreated water and foods. Unfortunately, one side effect to this lifestyle has been some increases in giardiasis as well as exposure to other amebic diseases. On the other hand, affluence has many benefits. Home freezers contribute to the control of trichinosis, because freezing pork for 6 days at 20°F will kill encysted larvae. Similarly, freezing foodstuffs for various time periods can prevent other diseases. In addition, use of window screens in more affluent countries is greatly reducing human exposure to disease-carrying vectors. The most valuable invention, however, for preventing the spread of parasitic infections has been the flush toilet, and its use everywhere is accompanied by decrease in disease. Probably the most effective control measure among our variety of measures may also be the hardest one to accomplish—the changing of human behavior through education and demonstrated rewards of improved health.

From the foregoing, it is evident that, on paper at least, parasitic diseases can be controlled by various methods, but until widespread control is achieved, a need will continue for chemotherapeutic intervention for infected individuals. Before treating a given infection with chemotherapy, the physician weighs several factors, including the severity and duration of infection, the health conditions of the host, and the availability and toxicity of the drug treatment. If the side effects or toxicity of a treatment will be more hazardous to the patient than the disease itself, then treatment may be reasonably withheld. Furthermore, if the chance of reinfection is great and the disease is mild, then treatment is probably questionable at best.

Once the decision to treat an infection has been made, consideration of the need to treat asymptomatic family members or others closely associated with the infected individual is important. For example, some parasites such as *Giardia* may be easily spread to others in a family or in an institutional setting, so treatment of other resident individuals may indeed be appropriate. Because *Trichomonas vaginalis* is transmitted sexually, all partners of the infected person should be treated as well. It is useless to treat others or isolate an infected person if direct transmission is not possible. This is why it is important to understand life cycles.

Some parasitic infections need not be treated because they are at a stage of low worm burdens, are self-limiting and nonpathogenic, and probably will not be transmitted to others. Some infections, however, require chemotherapy and/or surgical intervention. Cysticercosis and hydatid cysts at present require surgery, but treatment of amebiasis of the liver or appendix less often requires surgical attention, since more effective chemotherapeutics are now available. Promising new drugs are under study.

The objectives of a treatment program should be to stop the parasite's growth and reproduction, to kill parasites without inducing a harmful host response, and/or to expel parasites from the host. Finding those drugs that are selective for parasitic metabolic systems without adversely affecting human systems has been difficult. Not surprisingly, many drugs are rather toxic, especially the ones that affect energy metabolism. A variety of drugs currently in use are known carcinogens or teratogens.

Most drugs commonly used to treat infections affect various metabolic pathways such as energy metabolism, cell wall synthesis, protein synthesis, membrane function, nucleic acid synthesis, or co-factor synthesis. Several drugs affect neuromuscular systems of the helminths. The selective action of many antiprotozoal drugs results from either preferential absorption of the drug by the parasite or from the ability of the drug to discriminate between isofunctional targets in the host cells versus those in the parasitic cell. Little is known about the selective action of most antihelminthic chemicals.

Drug resistance develops when pathogenic organisms are able to metabolize the drug to an inactive form, to alter their permeability to the drug, to use a metabolic pathway not affected by the drug, to increase enzyme production in order to overcome the level of the drug being administered, or to change the drug's binding site target on or inside of the organism.

The extent to which each of the drug resistance factors mentioned affects the treatment of parasitic disease is not fully known. Alterations in permeability, drug-binding activity, and enzyme production all have been demonstrated for some parasites, with altered permeability being the single most common resistance mechanism. Changes with respect to binding activity and enzyme production can be genetically passed to offspring.

Table 8–1 contains a partial listing of chemotherapeutic agents commonly in use at the present time, along with some of their important side effects. The reader will find a further listing and updating of agents and side effects in the *Medical Letters* cited in the bibliography for this chapter.

Treatment of amebiasis caused by *Entamoeba histolytica* (see Item 11 on Table 8–1) depends upon the severity of the clinical symptoms and on the parasites' locations in the host. Debate over the treatment of asymptomatic carriers continues; however, when treated, the person is usually given diiodohydroxyquin or dioxanide furoate. When either mild or severe intestinal signs are evident, metronidazole plus diiodohydroxyquin is the treatment of choice. Extraintestinal amebiasis may be treated using metronidazole. Diiodohydroxyquin is also required when there is a concurrent bowel infection. Because newer drugs are less toxic, emetine is no longer considered the best treatment for extraintestinal amebiasis. However, the higher cost and limited availability of newer drugs in other parts of the world have perpetuated the use of emetine.

Infections with *Trichomonas vaginalis* in either sex are effectively treated with the oral medication metronidazole. This drug should not be taken by pregnant women, however. Topical preparations containing halogenated hydroxyquinolines are useful in relieving the symptoms of vaginitis but may not completely eliminate the parasite, since the preparation may not reach every organism. Other topical preparations are also available. Sexual partners should be treated simultaneously.

The treatment of helminths relies on the correct identification of the parasite involved. Generally, mebendazole and pyrantel pamoate are considered the drugs of choice in the treatment of most intestinal nematode infections. Thiabendazole is useful against cutaneous and visceral larval migrans and *Strongyloides stercoralis*. Niclosamide is effective against cestodes. Praziquantel is effective against all *Schistosoma* spp. and other flukes, while metrifonate or oxamniquine are suitable alternates for some schistosomes.

Treatment of filariasis is accomplished with diethylcarbamazine; however, some authorities recommend excision of the adult *Onchocerca* worm before treatment, since this drug will not kill the adult. An alternative treatment for onchocerciasis begins with a three-week course of diethylcarbamazine followed by suramin. Suramin will kill the adult worm. Further, antihistamines or corticosteroids may be needed to reduce the allergic (Mazotti) reaction to disintegrating microfilariae. Extreme caution is needed while treating onchocerciasis, since the allergic reaction may be fatal.

Early diagnosis and treatment of African trypanosomiasis is important because treatment after the central nervous system is involved is quite difficult. Suramin sodium is the drug of choice early on, but since it does not cross the blood-brain barrier, melarsoprol is needed for the late disease stages. Nifurtimox is most useful when treating *Trypanosoma cruzi* infections. All drugs for African trypanosomiasis are very toxic, and most should be administered during hospitalization.

The treatment of malaria follows two strategies—clinical cure and radical cure. A clinical cure is accomplished when symptoms are relieved and asexual parasites are eliminated from peripheral circulation. However, this treatment does not necessarily mean that all parasites have been eradicated from the body. Chloroquine phosphate is the drug of choice for treating all species of malaria sensitive to the drug—it will produce a clinical cure but will not completely eliminate the parasite from the host in those infections caused by relapsing species of malaria. A radical cure (elimination of secondary tissue schizonts) for *Plasmodium vivax* and *P. ovale* is accomplished using primaquine phosphate as the second course of treatment.

Travelers to endemic areas, including former residents who are returning after living in nonmalarious areas for some time, are advised to begin taking chloroquine phosphate 1 to 2 weeks prior to departure, continue throughout their stay in the endemic area, and for 6 weeks after return. In addition, primaquine phosphate should be taken for two weeks after leaving the area. This prophylactic course will normally prevent disease. Since chloroquine phosphate does not prevent liver invasion by the parasite, it is especially important to use primaquine to prevent a relapse with *P. vivax* or *P. ovale*.

Various strains of *P. falciparum* have become resistant to chloroquine. Successful treatment of these infections requires the use of alternative antimalarials such as a combination of pyrimethamine and sulfadoxine. Quinine may be used in place of chloroquine phosphate.

For prophylaxis, the Centers for Disease Control recommend using sulfadoxine (500 mg) plus pyrimethamine (25 mg) PLUS chloroquine (300 mg) once weekly for travelers in endemic areas of resistant malaria. It should be noted that areas of chloroquine-resistant malaria are no longer limited to East Africa but now include many locations in central Africa as well.

There has been a high number of cases of parasitic infections reported in immunocompromised patients. The most likely patient population, growing in number, is the AIDS (acquired immunodeficiency syndrome) group. As of early 1988, over 53,000 cases of this viral infection were reported in the United States. AIDS cases reported from 99 countries of the world have been estimated to be over 150,000 in early 1988. The total is expected to reach over 1 million cases by 1991, with over 150,000 cases in the United States of which 50,000 new cases may occur annually.

The populations at risk are as follows:

1. IV drug users
2. Homosexual/bisexual men

3. Persons who received blood transfusions between 1978 and 1985
4. Prostitutes
5. Hemophiliacs
6. Persons seeking treatment for sexually transmitted diseases
7. Persons having multiple sexual partners
8. Persons who consider themselves at risk
9. Children born of infected mothers

There are four parasitic infections commonly seen in the AIDS patients. All four are protozoa: *Pneumocystis carinii* (pneumonia), *Toxoplasma gondii* (encephalitis), *Cryptosporidium* spp. (enterocolitis), and *Isospora belli* (enterocolitis). *Pneumocystis* and *Toxoplasma* are rather frequent, whereas *Cryptosporidium* and *Isospora* are much less frequent and usually associated with chronic diarrhea and chronic wasting syndrome ("slim disease"). The diagnosis of *Pneumocystis carinii* pneumonia (PCP) can be presumptive or confirmatory.

Expectorated sputum, bronchoscopy specimen, or open lung biopsy can be stained and evaluated for *Pneumocystis*. Treatment is a rather involved process as the patients frequently have adverse reactions to medications (trimethoprim-sulfamethoxazole or pentamidine isothionate).

Toxoplasmosis can be localized by computerized axial tomography (CAT) scan of the brain showing enhancing mass lesions (a white ring around the mass demonstrated with contrast dye). The diagnosis can be confirmed by histological examination of the lesion following brain biopsy. Treatment consists of pyrimethamine and sulfadiazine. Also, life-long maintenance therapy is frequently required.

Cryptosporidium and *Isospora* are diagnosed by evaluating a flotation concentration of feces and staining. *Cryptosporidium* is difficult to treat, requiring fluid replacement, nutrition and antidiarrheal medication. Spiramycin and eflornithine have given limited success. *Isospora* infections are treated with trimethoprim-sulfamethoxazole for approximately 1 month.

Treatment of parasitic diseases relies heavily on accurate diagnosis followed by good judgment on the part of the physician. Factors such as drug toxicity, the parasite's location in the host, the length of the treatment course, the way the drug may be administered, and the general condition of the patient, all must be considered in order to provide maximum benefit. If only one drug is available, however, and the patient's condition necessitates treatment, there may be no other choice. Furthermore, certain long treatment schedules may facilitate parasitic resistance to the drug or create cumulative toxicity problems for the patient. Finally, good nutritional management is important to help the patient overcome infection and promote resistance to subsequent infections. Note that some drugs are teratogenic in animals, and special care should be taken to avoid prescribing them to pregnant women. (Teratogens are noted in Table 8–1.)

TABLE 8–1. Chemotherapy of Parasitic Diseases

Infecting Organism	Disease	Chemotherapeutic Agent	Adverse Reactions*
Acanthamoeba spp.	Meningoencephalitis	sulfadiazine and flucytosine (experimental)	**Rash,** photosensitivity, hepatic and renal toxicity, blood dyscrasia, vasculitis
Ancylostoma brazilienses	Cutaneous larval migrans; creeping eruption	thiabendazole	**Nausea, vomiting, vertigo, rash,** leukopenia, color vision disturbance, tinnitus, shock

TABLE 8–1. *Continued*

Infecting Organism	Disease	Chemotherapeutic Agent	Adverse Reactions*
Ancylostoma duodenale	Hookworm	mebendazole or pyrantel pamoate	**GI disturbance** **GI disturbance,** dizziness, rash, fever
Ascaris lumbricoides	Roundworm	1. mebendazole or pyrantel pamoate 2. piperazine citrate	**GI disturbance** **GI disturbance,** dizziness, rash, fever **GI disturbance**
Balantidium coli	Balantidiasis	tetracycline or iodoquinol or metronidazole	**Anorexia, nausea, vomiting,** renal and hepatic impairment **Iodine toxicoderma,** rash, slight thyroid enlargement, nausea **Nausea, headache,** vomiting, diarrhea, vertigo, insomnia, ataxia
Clonorchis sinensis	Chinese liver fluke	praziquantel	Sedation, abdominal discomfort, fever, sweating, nausea, eosinophilia, photosensitivity, urticaria, vomiting, and diarrhea
Dientamoeba fragilis	Amebiasis	diiodohydroxy-quin or tetracycline or paromomycin	**Iodine toxicoderma,** rash, slight thyroid enlargement, nausea **Anorexia, nausea, vomiting,** renal and hepatic impairment **GI disturbance**
Diphyllo-bothrium latum	Fish tapeworm	niclosamide or praziquantel	Nausea, abdominal pain Sedation, abdominal discomfort, fever, sweating, nausea, eosinophilia, photosensitivity,

TABLE 8–1. Continued

Infecting Organism	Disease	Chemotherapeutic Agent	Adverse Reactions*
			urticaria, abdominal pain, vomiting, and diarrhea
		or paromomycin	**GI disturbance**
Dracunulus medinensis	Filariasis; guinea	1. Ivermectin 2. niridazole	**Immunosuppression, vomiting, cramps,** dizziness, headache
		or metronidazole	**Nausea, headache,** vomiting, diarrhea, vertigo, insomnia, ataxia
		or thiabendazole	**Nausea, vomiting, vertigo, rash,** leukopenia, color vision disturbance, tinnitus, shock
Echinococcus spp.	Hydatid cyst	mebendazole or albendazole	**GI disturbance**
Entamoeba histolytica	Amebiasis	diiodohyroxyquin	**Iodine toxicoderma,** rash, slight thyroid enlargement, nausea
	Intestinal disease	metronidazole	**Nausea, headache,** vomiting, diarrhea, vertigo, insomnia, ataxia
		plus diiodohyroxyquin	**Iodine toxicoderma,** rash, slight thyroid enlargement, nausea
	Hepatic disease	metronidazole	**Nausea, headache,** vomiting, diarrhea, vertigo, insomnia, ataxia
		or chloroquine plus	Vomiting, headache, pruritus, ocular damage, convulsions, psychosis, rash, hair, nail and mucous membrane discoloration

TABLE 8–1. *Continued*

Infecting Organism	Disease	Chemotherapeutic Agent	Adverse Reactions*
Enterobius vermicularis	Pinworm	pyrantel pamoate	**GI disturbance,** dizziness, rash, fever
		or mebendazole	**GI disturbance**
Fasciola hepatica	Liver rot; sheep liver fluke	bithionol†	Photosensitivity skin reaction, vomiting, diarrhea, abdominal pain, urticaria
		or praziquantel	Sedation, abdominal discomfort, fever, sweating, nausea, eosinophilia, photosensitivity, urticaria, abdominal pain, vomiting, and diarrhea
Fasciolopsis buski	Facioliasis	praziquantel	Sedation, abdominal discomfort, fever, sweating, nausea, eosinophilia, photosensitivity, urticaria, abdominal pain, vomiting, and diarrhea
		or niclosamide	Nausea, abdominal pain
		or tetrachloroethylene	**Epigastric burning, dizziness, headache**
Giardia lamblia	Giardiasis	quinacrine	Vomiting, vertigo, headache, psychosis, blood dyscrasia, ocular damage, rash, hepatic necrosis
		or metronidazole	**Nausea, headache, vomiting,** diarrhea, vertigo, insomnia, ataxia

TABLE 8–1. *Continued*

Infecting Organism	Disease	Chemotherapeutic Agent	Adverse Reactions*
		or furazolidone	**Nausea, vomiting**
Hymenolepis nana	Dwarf tapeworm	1. praziquantel	Sedation, abdominal discomfort, fever, sweating, nausea, eosinophilia, photosensitivity, urticaria, abdominal pain, vomiting, and diarrhea
		2. niclosamide	Nausea, abdominal pain
Heterophyes heterophyes	Heterophyiasis, intestinal fluke	praziquantel	Sedation, abdominal discomfort, fever, sweating, nausea, eosinophilia, photosensitivity, urticaria, abdominal pain, vomiting, and diarrhea
Isospora belli	Intestinal disease	trimethoprim-sulfamethoxazole (teratogenic in animals)	**Rash,** photosensitivity, hepatic and renal toxicity, blood dyscrasia, vasculitis
Leishmania braziliensis or *L. mexicana*	Leishmaniasis: mucocutaneous	1. antimony Na gluconate (Stibogluconate sodium) 2. amphotericin B	Muscle pain and joint stiffness, bradycardia, colic, diarrhea, rash **Chills, sweating, fever, muscle pain, abdominal pain, nausea, vertigo**
L. donovani	Leishmaniasis: visceral	1. antimony Na gluconate 2. pentamidine isethionate	Muscle pain and joint stiffness, bradycardia, colic, diarrhea, rash **Hypotension, hypoglycemia, vomiting, blood**

TABLE 8–1. *Continued*

Infecting Organism	Disease	Chemotherapeutic Agent	Adverse Reactions*
			dyscrasias, renal damage, rash, hepatic toxicity
L. tropica	Leishmaniasis: cutaneous	1. antimony Na gluconate	Muscle pain and joint stiffness, bradycardia, colic, diarrhea, rash
Loa loa	Filariasis; eyeworm	2. local heat Diethylcarbam-azine	**Allergic and febrile reactions** due to worm
Metagonimus yokogawai	Metagonimiasis; intestinal fluke	praziquantel or	Sedation, abdominal discomfort, fever, sweating, nausea, eosinophilia, photosensitivity, urticaria, abdominal pain, vomiting and diarrhea
		tetrachloro-ethylene	**Epigastric burning, dizziness, headache,** drowsiness, Antabuse-like effect with alcohol
Naegleria fowleri	Primary meningoencephalitis	amphotericin B	**Chills, sweating, fever, muscle pain, abdominal pain, nausea, vertigo**
Necator americanus	Hookworm	mebendazole or pyrantel pamoate	**GI disturbance** **GI disturbance,** headache, dizziness, rash, fever
Onchocerca volvulus	Filariasis; river-blindness	1. Ivermectin 2. diethylcarbam-azine plus suramin	**Allergic and febrile reactions** due to worm **Rash, pruritus, paresthesias, vomiting,** peripheral neuropathy, shock
Opisthorchis viverrini	Opisthorchiasis; liver fluke	praziquantel	Sedation, abdominal discomfort, fever,

TABLE 8–1. *Continued*

Infecting Organism	Disease	Chemotherapeutic Agent	Adverse Reactions*
			sweating, nausea, eosinophilia, photosensitivity, urticaria, abdominal pain, vomiting and diarrhea
Paragonimus westermani	Paragonimiasis; lung fluke	1. praziquantel	Sedation, abdominal discomfort, fever, sweating, nausea, eosinophilia, photosensitivity, urticaria, abdominal pain, vomiting and diarrhea
		2. bithionol	Photosensitivity skin reaction, vomiting, diarrhea, abdominal pain, urticaria
Pediculus humanus var. *corporus* or *capitus*	Lice	1. permethrin	Irritation to skin, eyes, and mucous membranes
		2. pyrethrins with piperonyl butoxide or 0.5% malathion lotion or 1% lindane	Irritation to skin, eyes, mucous membranes; ragweed-sensitized persons should not use
Plasmodium falciparum	Malignant malaria (chloroquine susceptible)	chloroquine phosphate N.B.: No primaquine after infection	Headache, vomiting, confusion, skin eruptions, retinal injury
	(chloroquine resistant)	quinine sulfate and	**Cinchonism, hypotension, arrhythmias,** blood dyscrasia, photosensitivity, blindness
		pyrimethamine plus	**Folic acid deficiency,** blood dyscrasia, rash, vomiting, convulsions, shock

TABLE 8–1. *Continued*

Infecting Organism	Disease	Chemotherapeutic Agent	Adverse Reactions*
	(comatose patient)	sulfadiazine or quinine and tetracycline	**Rash,** photosensitivity, hepatic and renal toxicity, blood dyscrasia, vasculitis
		Quinine (parenteral)	**Cinchonism, hypotension, arrhythmias,** blood dyscrasia, photosensitivity, blindness
Plasmodium malariae	Quartan malaria	chloroquine phosphate N.B.: No primaquine after infection	Headache, vomiting, confusion, skin eruptions, retinal injury
Plasmodium ovale	Ovale malaria	chloroquine phosphate	Headache, vomiting, confusion, skin eruptions, retinal injury
		followed by primaquine phosphate (prevents relapses)	**Hemolytic anemia** in G-6-PD-deficient patients, neutropenia, nausea, hypertension. Do not use during pregnancy.
Plasmodium vivax	Tertian malaria	chloroquine phosphate	Headache, vomiting, confusion, skin eruptions, retinal injury
		followed by primaquine phosphate (prevents relapses)	**Hemolytic anemia** in G-6-PD-deficient patients, neutropenia, nausea, hypertension. Do not use during pregnancy.
Pneumocystis carinii	Pneumocystosis	trimethoprim-sulfamethoxazole or	**Rash,** photosensitivity, hepatic and renal toxicity, blood dyscrasia, vasculitis
		pentamidine isethionate	**Breathlessness, dizziness, headache,** tachycardia, vomiting, itching

TABLE 8–1. *Continued*

Infecting Organism	Disease	Chemotherapeutic Agent	Adverse Reactions*
Pthirus pubis	Crab lice	0.5% malathion lotion or 1% lindane	Irritation of skin, eyes, mucous membranes; ragweed-sensitized persons should not use
Sarcoptes scabiei	Mites; scabies	1. 1% lindane 2. 10% crotamiton	Irritation of skin, eyes, and mucous membranes, allergic reactions
Schistosoma haematobium	Schistosomiasis; bladder worm	praziquantel	Sedation, abdominal discomfort, fever, sweating, nausea, eosinophilia
Schistosoma japonicum	Schistosomiasis; blood fluke	praziquantel	Sedation, abdominal discomfort, fever, sweating, nausea, eosinophilia
Schistosoma mansoni	Schistosomiasis; blood fluke; swamp fever	praziquantel or	Sedation, abdominal discomfort, fever, sweating, nausea, eosinophilia
		oxamniquine (Vansil)	Headache, fever, dizziness, nausea, insomnia, diarrhea, hepatic enzyme changes
Strongyloides stercoralis	Threadworm	thiabendazole	**Nausea, vomiting, vertigo, rash,** leukopenia, color vision disturbance, tinnitus, shock
Taenia saginata	Cestode; beef tapeworm	1. niclosamide	Nausea, abdominal pain
		2. praziquantel	Sedation, abdominal discomfort, fever, sweating, nausea, eosinophilia, photosensitivity, urticaria, abdominal pain, vomiting, and diarrhea

TABLE 8–1. *Continued*

Infecting Organism	Disease	Chemotherapeutic Agent	Adverse Reactions*
Taenia solium	Cestode; pork tapeworm	1. niclosamide	Nausea, abdominal pain
		2. praziquantel	Sedation, abdominal discomfort, fever, sweating, nausea, eosinophilia, photosensitivity, urticaria, abdominal pain, vomiting, and diarrhea
	cysticercosis	1. praziquantel (experimental)	Sedation, abdominal discomfort, fever, sweating, nausea, eosinophilia, photosensitivity, urticaria, abdominal pain, vomiting, and diarrhea
		2. (surgery)	
Toxocara canis	Visceral larval migrans	1. thiabendazole	**Nausea, vomiting, vertigo, rash,** leukopenia, color vision disturbance, tinnitus, shock
		or diethylcarbam-azine	**GI disturbance**
		2. mebendazole	**GI disturbance**
Toxoplasma gondii	Toxoplasmosis (moderate–severe illness)	1. pyrimethamine and	**Folic acid deficiency,** blood dyscrasia, rash, vomiting, convulsions, shock; administer corticosteroids in ocular toxoplasmosis
		trisulfapyrimidines	**Rash,** photosensitivity, hepatic and renal toxicity
		(teratogenic in animals)	Blood dyscrasia, vasculitis
		2. spiramycin	GI disturbance

TABLE 8–1. *Continued*

Infecting Organism	Disease	Chemotherapeutic Agent	Adverse Reactions*
	(Immunosuppressed host)	pyrimethamine and	**Folic acid deficiency,** blood dyscrasia, rash, vomiting, convulsions, shock; administer corticosteroids in ocular toxoplasmosis
		sulfadiazine plus folinic acid	**Rash,** photosensitivity, hepatic and renal toxicity, blood dyscrasia, vasculitis
Trichinella spiralis	Trichinosis	thiabendazole and/or prednisone	**Nausea, vomiting, vertigo, rash,** leukopenia, color vision disturbance, tinnitus, shock
Trichomonas vaginalis	Trichomoniasis	metronidazole or benznidazole	**Nausea, headache, vomiting,** diarrhea, vertigo, insomnia, ataxia
Trichuris trichiura	Whipworm	mebendazole	**GI disturbance**
Trypanosoma cruzi	Chagas' disease	nifurtimox†	Nausea, dizziness, insomnia, peripheral neuropathy
Trypanosoma gambiense	West African sleeping sickness Hemolymphatic disease	1. suramin†	**Rash, pruritus, vomiting, paresthesias,** shock, peripheral neuropathy
		2. pentamidine isthionate	**Breathlessness, dizziness, headache,** tachycardia, vomiting, itching
	CNS disease	melarsoprol	**Encephalopathy,** vomiting, neuropathy, rash, myocarditis, hypertension
Trypanosoma rhodesiense	East African sleeping sickness	1. suramin†	**Rash, pruritus, vomiting,**

TABLE 8–1. *Continued*

Infecting Organism	Disease	Chemotherapeutic Agent	Adverse Reactions*
	Hemolymphatic disease		**paresthesias,** shock, peripheral neuropathy
		2. pentamidine isthionate	**Breathlessness, dizziness, headache,** tachycardia, vomiting, itching
	CNS disease	1. melarsoprol	**Encephalopathy,** vomiting, neuropathy, rash, myocarditis, hypertension
		2. tryparsamide and suramin†	**Nausea, vomiting** **Rash, pruritus, vomiting, paresthesias,** shock, peripheral neuropathy
Wuchereria bancrofti	Filariasis; Bancroft's filaria	diethylcarbamazine	**Allergic and febrile reactions** due to worm

*Most frequent adverse reactions to chemotherapy are noted in **boldface.**
†Available from CDC Drug Service, Centers for Disease Control, Atlanta, GA 30333.

BIBLIOGRAPHY

ALTMAN, RM, KEMAN, CM, AND BORCHAM, MM: *An outbreak of culicoides guyensis in the Canal Zone.* Mosquito News 30(2):231–235, 1970.

ALTMAN, RM, ET AL: *Control of Culicoides sand flies, Fort Kobbe Canal Zone in 1968.* Mosquito News 30(2):235–240, 1970.

CENTERS FOR DISEASE CONTROL: *Update: Chloroquin-Resistant Plasmodium falciparum-Africa.* MMWR 32(33):437–438, 1983.

CENTERS FOR DISEASE CONTROL: Revised recommendations for preventing malaria in travelers to areas with chloroquine-resistant *Plasmodium* falciparum. MMWR 14(4):185–190, 1985.

COX, FEG (ED): *Modern Parasitology: A Textbook of Parasitology.* Blackwell Scientific Publications, St Louis, 1982.

The Medical Letter, January 31, 1986.

The Medical Letter, February 12, 1988.

PAMPANO, E: *A Textbook of Malaria Eradication.* Oxford University Press, London, 1963.

PEARSON, R, GUERRANT, R: *Praziquantel: A major advance in antihelminthic therapy.* Annals of Internal Medicine 99, p 195, 1983.

Physicians Desk Reference, ed 42. Medical Economics Company, Oradell, NJ, 1988.

Proceedings of a Symposium of the International Atomic Energy Commission: Sterile insect technique and radiation in insect control. June 29–July 3, 1981, United Nations, New York, 1982.

SCHULTZ, MG: *Current Concepts in Parasitology: Parasitic Diseases.* N Engl J Med 297:1259–1261, 1977.

SOULSBY, EJL: *Immune Responses in Parasitic Infections: Immunology, Immunopathology and Immunoprophylaxis* (4 Vols). CRC Press, Boca Raton, FL, 1986.

WYNGAARDEN, LB AND SMITH, LH: *Cecil Textbook of Medicine,* ed 16. WB Saunders, Philadelphia, 1982.

FINAL EXAMINATION

Using separate sheets of paper, answer the following questions. Allow 90 minutes to complete this test. **Except when indicated, all questions are worth 1 point each.** A satisfactory score is 80 percent or more. Answers are given in the next section.

1. State the scientific name for the parasites illustrated below. (*5 points*).

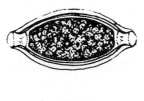

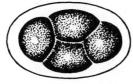

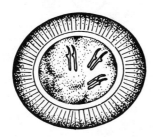

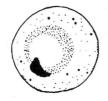

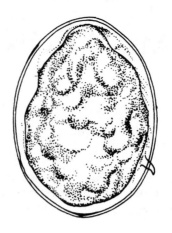

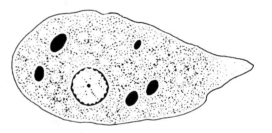

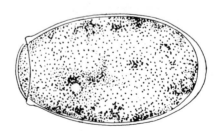

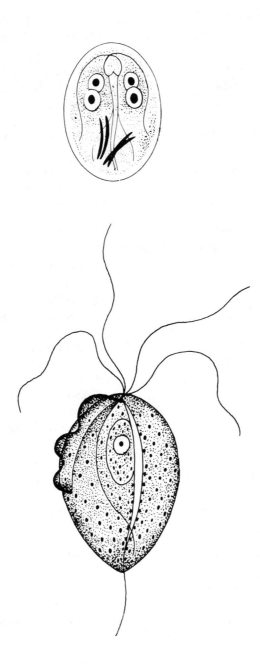

2. Draw the life cycle for each parasite given below. (**10 points**)

   a. *Ascaris lumbricoides*   d. *Enterobius vermicularis*
   b. *Diphyllobothrium latum*   e. *Leishmania donovani*
   c. *Trypanosoma cruzi*

3. A patient was treated with immunosuppressants during a kidney transplant and subsequently exhibited symptoms of two parasitic infections. Which were they? (**2 points**)

   a. *Ascaris lumbricoides*   d. *Strongyloides stercoralis*
   b. *Toxoplasma gondii*   e. *Plasmodium falciparum*
   c. *Schistosoma mansoni*

4. Which one of the following parasites is *not* found most prevalently in North or South America?

   a. *Trypansoma cruzi*   d. *Mansonella ozzardi*
   b. *Leishmania braziliensis*   e. *Paragonimus westermani*
   c. *Necator americanus*

5. For each parasite given, select its most common body location in humans. Choices may be used more than once. (**5 points**).

   a. _10_ *Schistosoma mansoni*   1. blood
   b. _2_ *Clonorchis sinensis*   2. liver
   c. _3_ *Trichura trichiura*   3. intestine
   d. _11_ *Leishmania braziliensis*   4. striated muscle
   e. _1_ *Trypanosoma rhodesiense*   5. skin
   f. _2_ *Echinococcus granulosus*   6. lymph nodes
   g. _3_ *Endolimax nana*   7. heart muscle
   h. _1_ *Plasmodium vivax*   8. eye
   i. _3_ *Strongyloides stercoralis*   9. bladder veins
   j. _2_ *Loa loa*   10. intestinal veins
                                        11. subcutaneous tissue
                                        12. macrophages

6. The intermediate host for Taenia saginata is

   a. pig   d. bear
   b. cow   e. sheep
   c. man

7. Which of the following are the diagnostic morphologic characteristics for *Entamoeba histolytica*?

   a. centrally located karyosome   e. large karyosome with a faintly visible
   b. a micro- and macro-nucleus   nuclear membrane
   c. large glycogen vacuole   f. ingested red blood cells
   d. flagella

8. Which of the following require no intermediate host?

   a. *Hymenolepis nana*   d. *Trichuris trichiura*
   b. *Giardia lamblia*   e. *Schistosoma mansoni*
   c. *Strongyloides stercoralis*

9. Which cestode produces an operculated egg?

   a. *Taenia saginata*   d. *Echinococcus granulosus*
   b. *Hymenolepis nana*   e. *Taenia solium*
   c. *Diphyllobothrium latum*

10. A stained blood smear reveals giant platelets and many reticulocytes containing Schuffner's dots, large ring forms, and schizonts with 12–24 merozoites. You would name this as

   a. *Plasmodium vivax*
   b. *Plasmodium falciparum*
   c. *Plasmodium ovale*
   d. *Plasmodium malariae*
   e. *Babesia* spp.

11. When purged specimens are to be examined for amebae, which of the following should be used to obtain the specimen?

   a. barium salts
   b. castor oil
   c. Fleet's Phospho-Soda
   d. mineral oil

12. A stained fecal smear reveals mononucleate flagellates with a comma-shaped posterior, and lemon-shaped mononucleate cysts with a clear, nipple-like bleb at one end. You would name this as

   a. *Trichomonas hominis*
   b. *Chilomastix mesnili*
   c. *Trichomonas vaginalis*
   d. *Giardia lamblia*
   e. *Endolimax nana*

13. Infection with *Brugia malayi* is best diagnosed by

   a. zinc-sulfate flotation concentration
   b. cellophane tape test
   c. xenodiagnosis
   d. trichrome staining of a fecal smear
   e. Knott's concentration test

14. All but one of the following are methods of human infection with *Toxoplasma gondii*. Which of the following is *not* a method of toxoplasmosis infection?

   a. mosquito bite
   b. in-utero transmission
   c. ingestion of öocyst
   d. ingestion of pseudocyst in meat
   e. ingestion of trachyzoite in milk

15. Which of the following conditions is *not* a zoonotic infection?

   a. scabies
   b. swimmer's itch
   c. tropical eosinophilic lung
   d. visceral larval migrans
   e. cutaneous larval migrans

16. Patient traveled last summer to Africa and has a spiking fever every third day. A stained blood smear reveals

   a. *Plasmodium vivax*
   b. *Plasmodium malariae*
   c. *Plasmodium falciparum*
   d. *Plasmodium ovale*

17. Cercariae of this parasite penetrate the skin of humans, thereby causing infection.

   a. *Fasciolopsis buski*
   b. *Heterophyes heterophyes*
   c. *Schistosoma japonicum*
   d. *Paragonimus westermani*

18. These two infections were found by stool examination of a child who had a history of eating dirt. (*2 points*)

   a. *Trichinella spiralis*
   b. *Ascaris lumbricoides*
   c. *Paragonimus westermani*
   d. *Trichuris trichiura*
   e. *Taenia solium*

19. Recovery in human feces of a 7-mm long gravid proglottid containing 8 lateral uterine branches indicates infection with

    a. *Hymenolepis nana*   d. *Taenia saginata*
    b. *Diphyllobothrium latum*   e. *Taenia solium*
    c. *Echinococcus granulosus*

20. This parasite was found in the blood smear of a patient who had a recent summer vacation in New England and reported many insect and tick bites.

    a. *Plasmodium vivax*   c. *Phthiris pubis*
    b. AIDS virus   d. *Babesia* spp.

21. Pinworm disease can be best diagnosed by using

    a. the formalin-ether concentration   c. a direct fecal smear preparation
       method   d. none of the above
    b. the cellophane tape test

22. A small operculated egg with a light bulb shape was found in the feces of a patient with liver abnormalities.

    a. *Fasciola hepatica*   c. *Fasciolopsis buski*
    b. *Paragonimus westermani*   d. *Clonorchis sinensis*

23. Mature trophozoites and young schizonts in blood smear show a distinct tendency toward band formation and the red blood cells are not enlarged.

    a. *Plasmodium vivax*   c. *Plasmodium falciparum*
    b. *Plasmodium malariae*   d. *Plasmodium ovale*

24. Found in the feces of a patient complaining of abdominal distress and diarrhea.

    a. *Giardia lamblia*   c. *Chilomastix mesnili*
    b. *Trichomonas vaginalis*   d. *Trichomonas tenax*

25. Only one of the following parasites produces eggs that are immediately infective to humans, and the eggs infect a person directly via ingestion. Which is it?

    a. *Schistosoma mansoni*   d. *Clonorchis sinensis*
    b. *Enterobius vermicularis*   e. *Taenia saginata*
    c. *Trichuris trichiura*

26. Match the arthropod vectors with the appropriate organism. (**5 points**)

    a. __5__ mosquito (*Culex* spp.)   1. *Loa loa*
    b. __2__ black fly (*Simulium* spp.)   2. *Onchocerca volvulus*
    c. __1__ mango fly (*Chrysops* spp.)   3. *Trypanosoma rhodesiense*
    d. __4__ crustacean (*Cyclops* spp.)   4. *Diphyllobothrium latum*
    e. __3__ tsetse fly (*Glossina* spp.)   5. *Wuchereria bancrofti*

27. Which of the following intestinal protozoa are *not* identified as a causative agent of diarrhea?

    a. *Entamoeba histolytica*   d. *Balantidium coli*
    b. *Dientamoeba fragilis*   e. *Entamoeba coli*
    c. *Giardia lamblia*

28. Identified from the bloody sputum of an immigrant from the Far East:

    a. *Fasciola hepatica*   c. *Paragonimus westermani*
    b. *Clonorchis sinensis*   d. *Fasciolopsis buski*

29. Control of a flea infestation is different from control of lice. Why?

    a. fleas are much more resistant to insecticides
    b. fleas reproduce off of the host, laying eggs in the environment
    c. fleas are larger than lice
    d. fleas don't need a blood meal

30. In clinical cases of *Wuchereria bancrofti,* the most favorable time to find parasites in the blood is

    a. early morning
    b. middle of the night
    c. during late afternoon
    d. anytime

31. Match the disease with the causative parasite. (***4 points***)

    a. ____ creeping eruption
    b. ____ visceral larval migrans
    c. ____ tropical eosinophilia
    d. ____ eosinophilic meningitis

    1. *Dirofilaria* spp.
    2. *Anasakis* spp.
    3. *Angiostrongylus* spp.
    4. *Toxocara* spp.
    5. *Ancylostoma caninum*

32. All of the following except one are best diagnosed by identification in a blood smear. Which one is not?

    a. *Trypanosoma gambiense*
    b. *Babesia microti*
    c. *Plasmodium falciparum*
    d. *Onchocerca volvulus*
    e. *Wuchereria bancrofti*

33. All of the following, except one, infect humans by entrance of the infective stage through the skin. Which one has a different route of entrance?

    a. *Schistosoma japonicum*
    b. *Strongyloides stercoralis*
    c. *Ancylostoma duodenale*
    d. *Necator americanus*
    e. *Heterophyes heterophyes*

34. Match the following with the appropriate statement. (***10 points***)

    1. *Entamoeba histolytica*
    2. *Entamoeba coli*
    3. *Endolimax nana*
    4. *Iodamoeba bütschlii*
    5. *Dientamoeba fragilis*

    a. ____ Which ameba trophozoite feeds on red blood cells?
    b. ____ Which ameba has a nucleus with a heavy chromatin ring and an eccentrically located karyosome?
    c. ____ Which ameba has a nucleus with an even chromatin ring and a centrally located karyosome?
    d. ____ Which ameba has up to four nuclei in a round cyst?
    e. ____ Which ameba cyst contains a glycogen vacuole?
    f. ____ Which ameba has a nucleus with a large karyosome and a chromatin ring that is not visible?
    g. ____ Which ameba does not form cysts?
    h. ____ Which ameba causes intestinal ulcers and bloody dysentery?
    i. ____ Which ameba can invade the liver and cause pathology in that organ?
    j. ____ Which ameba forms the smallest cyst?

35. The trichrome stain is used to identify

    a. blood protozoa
    b. helminth eggs in feces
    c. intestinal protozoa
    d. antibodies to tissue parasites

36. Below are listed sources of error that may have impact on a quality smear stained for parasites. Identify which one is *not* a source of error.

    a. blood smear too thick
    b. blood smear too new
    c. stain buffer has wrong pH
    d. wrong timing during staining

37. The head of scolex of *Diphyllobothrium latum*

    a. is armed with hooks
    b. has a retractable rostellum
    c. has four suckers
    d. has two sucking grooves

38. Egg has a large lateral spine.

    a. *Schistosoma haematobium*
    b. *Clonorchis sinensis*
    c. *Fasciola hepatica*
    d. *Schistosoma mansoni*

39. Which of the following is the best transport preservative for protozoan of flagellate trophozoites?

    a. zinc sulfate
    b. formalin and ether

    c. polyvinyl alcohol
    d. iodine

40. The cysticercus larva form is found where noted as part of the life cycle of which parasite?

    a. on aquatic vegetation; *Fasciola hepatica*
    b. in fish muscle; *Diphyllobothrium latum*
    c. in pork muscle; *Taenia solium*
    d. in mosquitoes; *Dracunculus medinensis*

41. Which of these Platyhelminthes infects humans through ingestion of undercooked fish? (You may choose more than one answer.) **(5 points)**

    a. *Clonorchis sinensis*
    b. *Paragonimus westermani*
    c. *Diphyllobothrium latum*

    d. *Heterophyes heterophyes*
    e. *Schistosoma mansoni*
    f. *Echinococcus granulosus*

42. *Babesia* spp. is transmitted to humans

    a. by the bite of an infected tick
    b. by the bite of an infected fly (*Chrysops* spp.)
    c. by ingestion of a cyst
    d. by the bite of an infected mosquito (*Anopheles* spp.)

43. Name two zoonotic infections caused by (**6 points**)

    a. nematodes
    b. protozoa
    c. platyhelminthes

44. Which of the following causes amebic meningoencephalitis?

    a. *Entamoeba histolytica*
    b. *Babesia* spp.
    c. *Naegleria* spp.

    d. *Sarcocystis* spp.
    e. *Acanthamoeba* spp.

45. Because you are responsible for parasite control on an island, you chemically treat the small freshwater lake for snails, but you accidently dump in too much chemical and kill every living thing in the lake. Your action breaks the life cycle and controls the spread of which of the following parasites? (Choose all correct answers.) (**5 points**)

    a. *Fasciolopsis buski*
    b. *Taenia solium*
    c. *Schistosoma mansoni*

    d. *Diphyllobothrium latum*
    e. *Hymenolepis nana*

46. Which of the following requires two different intermediate hosts in its life cycle?

    a. *Clonorchis sinensis*
    b. *Schistosoma mansoni*
    c. *Trichuris trichiura*

    d. *Loa loa*
    e. *Echinococcus granulosus*

47. Which of the following exhibits diurnal periodicity?

    a. *Wuchereria bancrofti*
    b. *Brugia malayi*

    c. *Loa loa*
    d. *Onchocerca volvulus*

48. Below is shown the final centrifuge tube appearance for two different concentration techniques. Indicate where the parasites are found in each tube and state what concentration techniques each tube represents. (**5 points**)

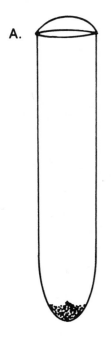

A.

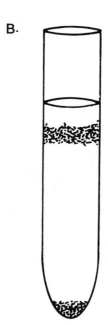

B.

Answer Key

CHAPTER 1 (PRE-TEST)

1. b
2. d
3. c
4. c
5. c
6. a
7. d
8. b
9. a
10. c
11. a = 3; b = 5; c = 1; d = 2; e = 4
12. a. vector: any arthropod or other living carrier that transports a pathogenic microorganism from an infected to a noninfected host.
    b. host: the species of animal or plant that harbors a parasite and provides some metabolic resources to the parasitic species.
    c. proglottid: one of the segments of a tapeworm; each contains male and female reproductive organs when mature.
    d. definitive host: animal in which a parasite passes its adult existence and/or sexual reproduction phase.
    e. operculum: the lid or caplike cover on certain helminth eggs.

CHAPTER 2

1.

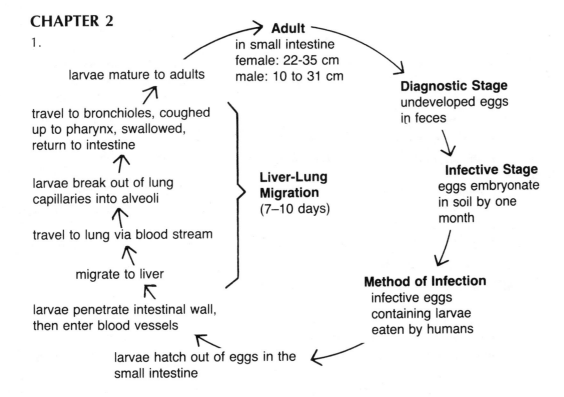

larvae mature to adults

travel to bronchioles, coughed up to pharynx, swallowed, return to intestine

larvae break out of lung capillaries into alveoli

travel to lung via blood stream

migrate to liver

larvae penetrate intestinal wall, then enter blood vessels

Liver-Lung Migration (7–10 days)

Adult
in small intestine
female: 22-35 cm
male: 10 to 31 cm

Diagnostic Stage
undeveloped eggs
in feces

Infective Stage
eggs embryonate
in soil by one
month

Method of Infection
infective eggs
containing larvae
eaten by humans

larvae hatch out of eggs in the small intestine

2. a. *Wuchereria bancrofti*
    b. *Culex* or *Anopheles* spp. mosquito
    c. blood specimen, stained thick and thin smears. Concentrate the specimen by centrifugation. Serology helpful also.

3. a. **cutaneous larval migrans.** A disease caused by the migration of larvae of *Ancylostoma* spp. (dog or cat hookworm) or other helminths under the skin of humans. Larval migration is marked by thin, red, papular lines of eruption. Also termed creeping eruption.
    b. **diurnal.** Occurring during the daytime.
    c. **diagnostic stage.** A developmental stage of the pathogenic organism that can be detected in human body secretions, discharges, feces, blood, or tissue by chemical means or microscopic observation as an aid in diagnosis.
    d. **infective stage.** The stage of a parasite at which it is capable of entering the host and continuing development within the host.
    e. **prepatent stage.** The time elapsing between initial infection with the parasite and reproduction by the mature parasite.

4.

Scientific Name	Common Name	Method of Infection	Body Specimen to Examine
Trichuris trichiura	whipworm	ingestion of developed eggs from soil	feces for eggs
Onchocerca volvulus	blinding filaria	black fly (simulium)	tissue scraping of nodule for microfilaria
Strongyloides stercoralis	threadworm	filariform larvae penetrates skin	feces for rhabditiform larvae; duodenal specimen for eggs.
Ancylostoma duodenale	Old World hookworm	filariform larvae penetrate skin	feces for eggs
Enterobius vermicularis	pinworm, seatworm	ingestion of developed eggs: hand to mouth from scratching perianal area	cellophane tape press of perianal area for eggs and adult

All these migrate in the lungs as larvae during infection:

5. *Ascaris lumbricoides*
    Trichinella spiralis
    Necator americanus
    Ancylostoma duodenale
    Strongyloides stercoralis

CHAPTER 3

1. a. **hexacanth embryo.** A tapeworm larva having six hooklets (see **onchosphere**); found in all *Taenia* spp. eggs.
    b. **hermaphroditic.** Having both male and female reproductive organs within the same individual. All tapeworms have both sets of reproductive organs in each segment of the adult (i.e., all adult tapeworms are hermaphroditic).

      c. **"armed" scolex.** Crown of hooks on anterior end of a tapeworm; causes attachment to the wall of the intestine of a host by means of suckers and hooks (e.g., *Taenia solium*).

      d. **proglottid.** One of the segments of a tapeworm (all adult tapeworms form proglottids). Each proglottid contains male and female reproductive organs when mature.

      e. **hydatid cyst.** A vesicular structure formed by *Echinococcus granulosus* larvae in the intermediate host; contains fluid, blood capsules, and also daughter cysts in which the scolices of potential tapeworms are formed.

2. a. 5 (4)
  b. 4
  c. 7
  d. 2,1
  e. 10 (4)

3. a. *Hymenolepis nana*

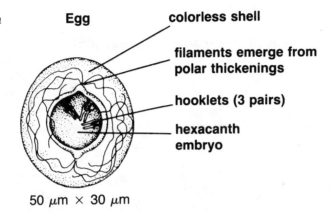

50 μm × 30 μm

  b. *Diphyllobothrium latum*

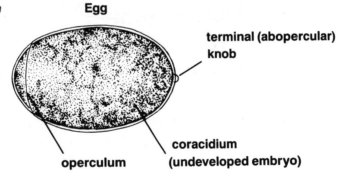

75 μm × 45 μm

  c. *Taenia saginata*

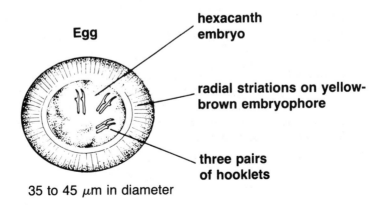

35 to 45 μm in diameter

d. *Taenia solium*

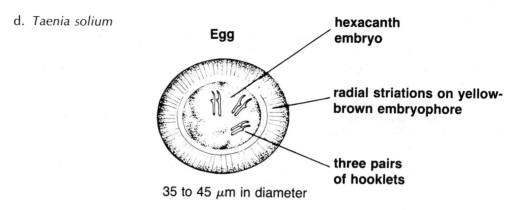

Egg

hexacanth
embryo

radial striations on yellow-
brown embryophore

three pairs
of hooklets

35 to 45 μm in diameter

e. *Echinococcus granulosus*

Hydatid cyst (partial cross-section)

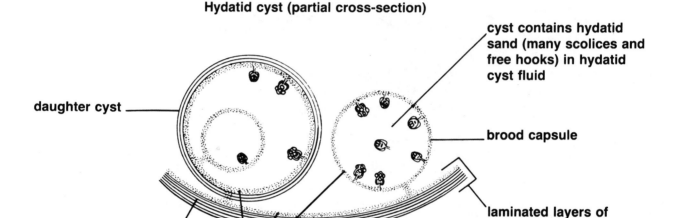

cyst contains hydatid
sand (many scolices and
free hooks) in hydatid
cyst fluid

daughter cyst

brood capsule

laminated layers of
inner germinal tissue
and outer covering

cyst wall

germinal layer

NOTE: Gravid proglottids and scolex are also diagnostic.

4. a. 6   e. 8
   b. 2   f. 7
   c. 5   g. 3
   d. 1   h. 4

CHAPTER 4

1. 1 egg   6 metacercaria   2 miracidium   4 redia
   7 adult   3 sporocyst   5 cercaria

2. D. Possible contact with sheep-, sheepdog-, and freshwater fish-transmitted parasites.
   a. no contact with pigs. No contact with snails or fish hosts of Oriental lung fluke
   b. no contact with snails which host *S. mansoni* or hosts of *C. sinensis*
   c. no contact with snail hosts of *S. japonicum*
   d. no contact with snails or fish hosts of *H. heterophyes*

3. a. 1. *Fasciolopsis buski* (large intestinal fluke), ingestion
      2. *clonorchis sinensis* (Chinese liver fluke)
      3. *Schistosoma mansoni* (Manson's blood fluke)
   b. 1. human eats metacercaria on uncooked water plant

2. human eats metacercaria on uncooked fish

3. cercaria penetrate skin

4. Method of infection with blood flukes (schistosomes) is by penetration of the skin by cercaria in fresh water. Prevention of infection with blood flukes therefore requires prohibiting human feces or urine from contaminating fresh water; snail control; root entering contaminated water without protection; treating carriers with drugs; and education.

Prevention of infection with intestinal flukes requires cooking all fish and crustaceans thoroughly; washing water plants such as watercress and water chestnuts thoroughly; education about method of infections as well as education about not contaminating fresh water with human waste; treating carriers; and snail control.

CHAPTER 5

1. a. 4   g. 2
   b. 7   h. 9,10
   c. 14   i. 1
   d. 8   j. 3
   e. 11   k. 6
   f. 5,1,2   l. 12

2. In trophozoite: study differential characteristics of size, consistency and inclusions (bacterial or red blood cells) in cytoplasm, directional vs. random motility, shape of pseudopods, staining characteristics of nuclear structures. In cysts: study differential characteristics of size, number of nucleii and nuclear structure, shape of chromotoidal bodies.

3. a. **trophozoite.** The motile stage of a protozoan which feeds, multiplies, and maintains the colony within the host.

   b. **cyst.** The immotile stage protected by a cyst wall formed by the parasite. In this stage, the protozoan is readily transmitted to a new host.

   c. **sporozoite.** The form of *Plasmodium* that develops inside the sporocyst, invades the salivary glands of the mosquito, and is transmitted to humans.

   d. **schizogony.** Asexual multiplication of *Apicomplexa*; multiple intracellular nuclear division precedes cytoplasmic division.

   e. **carrier.** A host harboring and disseminating a parasite but exhibiting no clinical signs or symptoms.

   f. **öocyst.** The encysted form of the öokinete; occurs on the stomach wall of *Anopheles* spp. mosquitoes infected with malaria.

   g. **pseudocyst.** A cystlike structure formed by the host during an acute infection with *Toxoplasma gondii*. The cyst is filled with tachyzoites in normal hosts; may occur in brain or other tissues. Latent source of infection which may become active if immunosuppression occurs.

   h. **L.D. body (Leishman-Donovan body).** Each of the small ovoid amastigote forms found in tissue macrophages of the liver and spleen in patients with *Leishmania donovani* infection.

   i. **paroxysm.** The fever-chills syndrome in malaria. Spiking fever corresponds to the release of merozoites and toxic materials from the parasitized red blood cell (RBC), and shaking chills occur during schizont development. Occurs in malaria cyclically every 36 to 72 hours, depending on the species.

   j. **atrium** (pl. **atria**). An opening; in a human, refers to the mouth, vagina, and urethra.

4. a. bite of *Phlebotomus* spp.

   b. ingestion of cyst in contaminated water or food

   c. infected feces of *Triatome* spp. rubbed into bite or conjunctiva

   d. ingestion of öocyst, trophozoite, or pseudocyst; congenital transmission

e. in men, sexual intercourse; in women, contamination with infectious material from vagina
f. ingestion of cyst in contaminated water or food
g. tick bite
h. bite of *Anopheles* mosquito; contaminated blood ingestion
i. bite of *Glossina* spp.
j. bite of *Phlebotomus* spp.

5. *P. vivax*

Trophozoite (single ring)

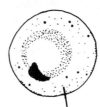

Schüffner's dots

**Note: Single ring, one third diameter of an RBC; invades only immature RBCs so that large bluish cells are parasitized.
RBC shows red-stained Schüffner's dots which become visible between 15 and 20 hours following invasion of the cell.**

P. malariae

Trophozoite (single ring)

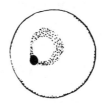

Note: Trophozoite forms band across RBC during early schizogony.

Trophozoites

P. falciparum

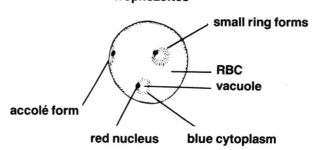

small ring forms

RBC
vacuole

accolé form

red nucleus   blue cytoplasm

CHAPTER 6

1. a. 5
   b. 6
   c. 1
   d. 3
   e. 2
2. a. 5   f. 3
   b. 1,2,3,4,5,7   g. 3
   c. 4   h. 1
   d. 6   i. 7
   e. 5   j. 3
3. All flea stages develop to maturity in the environment rather than on the host, as is the case with lice. Therefore, treatment for fleas must include chemically treating the

rooms of the house as well as the host. For lice, primary treatment is to the infected individual, although personal items such as combs, bedding, and towels must also be disinfected.

4. Annoyance, allergic reaction, blood loss, toxins or venom in bites, secondary bacterial infections, transmission of a variety of microorganisms by mechanical or biological methods, loss of food crops, loss of animal productivity, myiasis.

CHAPTER 7

1. False—1 or 2 is sufficient for helminths, 3 to 6 for suspected amebiasis or giardiasis.
2. True
3. False—not all intestinal protozoa form cysts; trophozoites die and hookworm eggs may hatch if specimen is not rapidly preserved.
4. True
5. False—oil enemas make examination impossible.
6. False—other species of parasites may also be present.
7. False—parasitemia may be too low. Thick smears are recommended in addition to thin smears.
8. Low light for contrast; unstained amebae are translucent.
9. First thing in the morning before washing or defecation because generally pinworms deposit eggs at night.
10. Formalin-ether; sedimentation of parasite stages. Zinc sulfate; flotation, based on differential specific gravity of parasites and the liquid media. For procedures, see pages 127–129.
11. 1.18 to 1.20; hydrometer
12. Schistosome eggs, infertile ascaris eggs, operculated eggs
13. Ether or ethyl acetate
14. Thin: little distortion, but hard to find the parasites. Thick: distortion, but easier to find parasites.
15. Place slide in distilled water until hemoglobin color disappears from slide.
16. Cytoplasm light blue-green or pink for *E. histolytica*, more purple for *E. coli*. Karyosomes stain ruby red.
17. Boeck-Drbohlav, Balamuth, Cleveland-Collier. Add sterile rice powder and stool to media. Incubate at 37°C for 24 hours; examine top of sediment for trophozoites.
18. Disodium phosphate and monosodium phosphate, ph 7.0
19. a. 2,4   f. 4
    b. 1,5   g. 8
    c. 6   h. 7
    d. 4   i. 4
    e. 3   j. 7

FINAL EXAMINATION

1. *Trichuris trichiuris*
   Necator americanus (or *Ancylostoma brazilienses*)
   Taenia solium or *Taenia saginata*
   Ascaris lumbricoides
   Plasmodium vivax
   Schistosoma japonicum
   Entamoeba histolytica
   Paragonimus westermani

Giardia lamblia
Trichomonis vaginalis

2. a = Diagram 2–4 (p 15); b = Diagram 3–3 (p 41); c = Diagram 5–6 (p 83); d = Diagram 2–2 (p 12); e = Diagram 5–7 (p 85).
3. b,d
4. e
5. a = 10; b = 2; c = 3; d = 12,5,11; e = 1; f = 2; g = 3; h = 1,(2); i = 3; j = 8,1
6. b
7. a,f
8. a,b,c,d
9. c
10. a
11. c
12. b
13. e
14. a
15. a
16. b
17. c
18. b,d
19. e
20. d
21. b
22. d
23. b
24. a
25. b
26. a = 5; b = 2; c = 1; d = 4; e = 3
27. e
28. c
29. b
30. b
31. a = 5; b = 4; c = 1; d = 3
32. d
33. e
34. a = 1; b = 2; c = 1; d = 1; e = 4; f = 3; g = 5; h = 1; i = 1; j = 3
35. c
36. b
37. d
38. d
39. c
40. c
41. a,c,d
42. a
43. a. *Ancylostoma* spp., *Angiostrongylus* spp., *Anisakis* spp., *Capillaria philippinensis*, *Dirofilaria* spp., *Gnathostoma* spp., *Gongylonema pulchrum*, *Thelasia* spp., *Toxocara* spp.
    b. *Trypanosoma* spp., *Sarcocystic* spp., *Leishmania* spp., *Toxoplasma gondii*, *Babesia* spp.
    c. *Fasciola hepatica*, swimmer's itch, *Echinococcus granulosus*, *Hymenolepis diminuta*, *Dipylidium caninum*, *Sparganosis*, *Cysticercosis*
44. e

45. a,c,d
46. a
47. c
48. a. parasites at the top of the fluid: flotation method
    b. parasites at the bottom of the tube: sedimentation method

INDEX

A page number in *italics* indicates a figure. A "*t*" following a page number indicates a table. A page number in **boldface** indicates a color plate.